Procedure
Coding

HANDBOOK FOR PSYCHIATRISTS

Fourth Edition

Procedure Coding

HANDBOOK FOR PSYCHIATRISTS

Fourth Edition

Chester W. Schmidt, Jr., M.D.
Rebecca K. Yowell
Ellen Jaffe

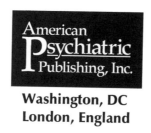

American Psychiatric Publishing, Inc.

Washington, DC
London, England

If you would like to buy between 25 and 99 copies of this or any other APPI title, you are eligible for a 20% discount; please contact APPI Customer Service at appi@psych.org or 800-368-5777. If you wish to buy 100 or more copies of the same title, please e-mail us at bulksales@psych.org for a price quote.

Manufactured in Canada on acid-free paper
14 13 12 11 10   5 4 3 2 1
Fourth Edition

Typeset in Adobe's Minion and Bitstream's Zapf Humanist.

American Psychiatric Publishing, Inc.
1000 Wilson Boulevard
Arlington, VA 22209-3901
www.appi.org

Library of Congress Cataloging-in-Publication Data
Schmidt, Chester W.
    Procedure coding handbook for psychiatrists / Chester W. Schmidt Jr., Rebecca K. Yowell, Ellen Jaffe. — 4th ed.
        p. ; cm.
    Rev. ed. of: CPT handbook for psychiatrists / Chester W. Schmidt Jr., Rebecca K. Yowell, Ellen Jaffe. 3rd ed. c2004.
    Includes bibliographical references and index.
    ISBN 978-1-58562-374-7 (pbk. : alk. paper)
    1. Physicians' current procedural terminology—Handbooks, manuals, etc. 2. Mental illness—Treatment—United States—Terminology—Handbooks, manuals, etc. 3. Mental illness—Treatment—United States—Code numbers—Handbooks, manuals, etc. I. Yowell, Rebecca, 1960– II. Jaffe, Ellen, 1946– III. Schmidt, Chester W. CPT handbook for psychiatrists. IV. Physician's current procedural terminology. V. Title.
    [DNLM: 1. Psychotherapy—classification—Terminology—English. 2. Forms and Records Control—Terminology—English. 3. Insurance Claim Reporting—Terminology—English. 4. Mental Disorders—classification—Terminology—English. 5. Relative Value Scales—Terminology—English. WM 15]
    RC465.6.S36 2011
    616.89001′2—dc22
                                                                            2010039455

British Library Cataloguing in Publication Data
A CIP record is available from the British Library.

Contents

About the Authors vii

Preface ix

Introduction xi

1 Basics of Current Procedural Terminology 1

2 Introduction to Documentation
of Psychiatric Services 7

3 Codes and Documentation for Psychiatric Services and
Other Mental Health Services 11

4 Codes and Documentation for Evaluation and
Management Services 29

5 Coding and Documentation for Specific Clinical Settings 63

6 Medicare 71

7 Commercial Insurance Issues 83

8 Putting It All Together for Accurate Coding 91

9 FAQs and Problem Scenarios 97

Appendixes

A   The CPT Coding System: How It Came to Be, How It Changes 101

B   The Health Insurance Portability and Accountability Act (HIPAA) 105

C   Modifiers. 111

D   Place of Service Codes for Medicare 113

E   1997 CMS Documentation Guidelines for Evaluation and Management
     Services (Abridged and Modified for Psychiatric Services). 115

F   Vignettes for Evaluation and Management Codes. 129

G   Most Frequently Missed Items in Evaluation and Management (E/M)
     Documentation 137

H   Documentation Templates 141

I   ECT Patient Information, Consent Form, and Record Template. 157

J   Examples of Relative Value Units (RVUs) (2010). 163

K   National Distribution of Evaluation and Management
     Code Selection by Psychiatrists 171

L   American Psychiatric Association CPT Coding Service and
     Additional Resources. 177

M   Medicare Carriers and Administrative Contractors 179

N   Centers for Medicare and Medicaid Services Regional Offices 181

Index 185

About the Authors

Chester W. Schmidt, Jr., M.D., is founding member of the American Medical Association (AMA) Relative Value Scale (RVS) Update Committee, consultant to the American Psychiatric Association (APA) RVS Update Committee, and professor of psychiatry at the Johns Hopkins University School of Medicine in Baltimore, Maryland.

Rebecca K. Yowell is deputy director of the APA Office of Healthcare Systems and Financing in Arlington, Virginia, and lead staff for APA's work with the AMA CPT Editorial Panel and AMA RVS Committee.

Ellen Jaffe is the Medicare specialist in the APA Office of Healthcare Systems and Financing in Arlington, Virginia, and is responsible for the Psychiatric Practice and Managed Care page that appears irregularly in *Psychiatric News.*

Preface

This fourth edition of the *Procedure Coding Handbook for Psychiatrists* marks more than a decade and a half of service to mental health practitioners. We hope this edition helps to further clarify the intricacies of coding and documentation for mental health services. Chapter 1 provides basic background information about Current Procedural Terminology (CPT) coding and describes the format of the current American Medical Association CPT manual so you'll know where to find things (for more in-depth information about the CPT Editorial Panel, which governs the CPT coding system, see Appendix A). Chapter 2 makes a case for complete and accurate documentation. Chapter 3 provides detailed descriptions of the psychiatric evaluation and therapeutic procedure codes as well as nonpsychiatric mental health services and explains how to document for each of them. In Chapter 4 you will find a discussion of the evaluation and management (E/M) codes, with an emphasis on the E/M codes used most frequently by mental health professionals, and an explanation of how to document for the E/M codes. Chapter 5, a new chapter, provides vignettes for different clinical sites and the coding solutions appropriate for these vignettes. Medicare issues are discussed in Chapter 6. Chapter 7 explores private health insurance and provides practical information about your relationship with these insurers. Chapter 8 is a summation of all that has come before. We have added another new chapter to this edition: Chapter 9, which provides frequently asked questions and problem scenarios based on queries that have come in through the American Psychiatric Association (APA) Managed Care Help Line.

The information in this book is the product of the collective experience and wisdom of the members of the Committee on RBRVS, Codes, and Reimbursements of the APA. The committee's principal mission is to monitor the work products and policies of the American Medical Association's CPT Editorial Panel and the RVS Update Committee to be able to inform and educate the APA membership about coding, documentation of services, and the Resource-Based Relative Value Scale (RBRVS) that is used by Medicare. All three of these elements directly affect every practitioners' reimbursement whether they are enrolled in Medicare or not. The committee sponsors workshops and courses at the APA's annual meeting. Members of the committee also provide workshops and lectures for APA district branches and state psychiatric societies. Academic medical centers, hospitals, and large group practices have received consultations from committee members as well. Whatever the format or venue, we have found that participants have readily expressed their need for assistance, and it is the concerns and questions they have brought to us over the years that have provided the framework for this edition of the handbook, just as they have for the previous three.

Members of the Committee on RBRVS, Codes, and Reimbursements— Ronald Burd, M.D.; Allan Anderson, M.D.; Naakesh Dewan, M.D.; Evan Eyler, M.D.; Jeffrey Feola, M.D.; Ed Gordon, M.D.; Tracy Gordy, M.D.; Jeremy Musher, M.D.; David Nace, M.D.; and Mark Russakoff, M.D.—all deserve acknowledgment for their contributions to this book. The leadership of Irvin "Sam" Muszynski, Director of the APA's Office of Healthcare Systems and Financing, as well as the support his staff provides, must also be acknowledged. Finally, thanks are due to Anita Everett, M.D., chair of the APA's Council on Healthcare Systems and Financing, for the extraordinary help she has provided to the committee.

Chester W. Schmidt, Jr., M.D.
Rebecca K. Yowell
Ellen Jaffe

Introduction

Both the regulatory climate and fiscal market in which mental healthcare is provided have continued to change since the first edition of this handbook was published in 1993. One would have hoped that by now, after more than 15 years of experience working with Current Procedural Terminology (CPT) codes and the Resource-Based Relative Value Scale (RBRVS), most mental health professionals would have a good working knowledge of procedural coding for psychiatric and evaluation and management services and of the attendant documentation requirements of the major payers. Unfortunately, although there has been much progress, our experience indicates there are still persistent gaps in knowledge about coding and documentation as well as questions about how to apply what is known to specific clinical settings.

Because of changes to the payment system, it is now more important than ever that clinicians be able to take advantage of the flexibility of the CPT coding system when coding for psychiatric services. Psychiatrists need to understand the use of the evaluation and management (E/M) codes as well as the psychiatry codes.

Using E/M codes rather than psychiatry codes, when appropriate, can have a significant impact on the level of reimbursement because of the different values attached to the codes. For instance, for inpatient work the psychiatry code 90801 (psychiatric diagnostic interview examination) is considered to be equivalent to the E/M code 99223 (initial hospital care, per day, for the evaluation and management of a patient). Although 90801 is valued at 3.53 relative value units (RVUs), which are used to calculate fees; 99223 is valued at 5.18 RVUs. This could mean a difference of more than $50 in payment for the same work.

It is vital that mental health clinicians understand that a legible, carefully constructed and documented medical record is essential to providing good patient care and that appropriate procedural coding is a necessary component of medical records keeping for both patient care and billing and collection activities. The medical record also serves additional purposes: documentation for services billed to patients; documentation of compliance with standards set by government agencies and insurance carriers; protection against audits by payers; and a source of evidence as to the "why, when, and how" of provided services in the case of a malpractice suit. Procedural coding is a necessary component of medical records keeping and of billing and collection activities.

The task of coding is complicated by the ongoing development of new treatment modalities and multiple sites of service (e.g., office, hospital, nursing home, partial hospital, assisted living facilities), and the American Medical Association (AMA) CPT manual is revised annually to reflect these changes. To code and document appropriately, the practitioner must have knowledge of the most current procedural codes and their supporting documentation requirements.

The American Psychiatric Association (APA) has always recognized the importance of accurate procedural coding. In the mid-1970s the association formed the CPT Coding Committee and, in collaboration with the AMA's CPT Editorial Panel, published two editions of *Procedural Terminology for Psychiatrists* (in 1975 and 1980). In 1988, the APA created the Work Group for Coding and Reimbursement, which became a standing committee in 1995. In 2001 this committee expanded its scope to become the Committee on RBRVS, Codes, and Reimbursements, reporting to the Council on Healthcare Systems and Financing.

The Committee on RBRVS, Codes, and Reimbursements is responsible for monitoring the activities of the AMA's CPT Editorial Panel; monitoring changes in Medicare's RBRVS payment system; representing psychiatry on the AMA Relative Value Scale (RVS) Update Committee; notifying other APA components when it is appropriate for them to assess modifications or additions to relevant CPT codes; initiating coding changes and modifications; and, most important, continually updating APA members about coding and documentation issues. Members of the committee are available to answer APA members' specific CPT coding questions. Questions must be in writing and should be sent to the CPT Coding Service at the APA's Office of Healthcare Systems and Financing by e-mail (hsf@psych.org), fax (703-907-1089), or regular mail (1000 Wilson Boulevard #1825, Arlington, VA 22209).

Committee members participate in the AMA RVS Update Committee and on the Advisory Committee of the Editorial Panel (see Appendix A). In recognition of the use of CPT by nonphysician mental health professionals, the committee also works collaboratively on coding and documentation issues with the American Psychological Association, the American Nurses Association, and the National Association of Social Workers.

Participation in the formal processes of CPT, the AMA RVS Update Committee, and with the Centers for Medicare and Medicaid Services, the federal agency that oversees Medicare, allows the committee to stay current on the issues of codes and reimbursement on an official level. The direct contact committee members have with APA members and other mental health professionals during courses and workshops and through the APA's Managed Care Help Line (800-343-4671 or hsf@psych.org) allows them to stay current with what is happening with codes and reimbursement on a day-to-day basis. Problems and questions that arise from practice experiences stimulate strategic thinking about coding, documentation, and reimbursement.

Mental health professionals continue to struggle with payers about the appropriate choice of codes for specific services and the relation of the code chosen to the level of reimbursement. Payers continue to challenge the "medical necessity" of services by denying the use of codes that have a higher reimbursement value. The fight for appropriate reimbursement goes on, with payers frequently using the technicalities of coding and documentation to reduce or deny payment. The committee takes very seriously its responsibility to provide support to practitioners in this ongoing struggle.

In large part, the purpose of this handbook is to equalize the playing field for practitioners and payers by enhancing the technical knowledge of practitioners about healthcare financing systems, codes, and documentation. The payers have their highly paid advisers to provide them with this support. To this end, the goals of this book are to provide an understanding of the structure and function of CPT, to provide an understanding of how to use the psychiatric therapeutic procedure codes and the E/M codes appropriate for psychiatric services and how to document for them, and to provide knowledge of the Medicare RBRVS payment system and how it affects the practice of psychiatry.

Basics of Current Procedural Terminology

Physicians' Current Procedural Terminology was first published by the American Medical Association (AMA) in 1966. The Current Procedural Terminology (CPT) coding system was created to provide a uniform language for describing medical and surgical procedures and diagnostic services that would facilitate more effective communication between clinicians, insurers, and patients. CPT 2010 represents a revision of the fourth edition of CPT, first published in 1977. A revision to the current edition is published every year.

The AMA's CPT Editorial Panel has the sole authority to revise, update, or modify CPT. The panel is composed of 15 physicians and 1 doctor of podiatric medicine. Ten of the physicians are nominated by the AMA, one of whom is appointed chair, and one member each is nominated by the American Hospital Association, the Blue Cross/Blue Shield Association, the Health Insurance Association of America, the AMA Healthcare Professionals Advisory Committee (composed of nonphysician members of the CPT Advisory Committee), and the Centers for Medicare and Medicaid Services. In 1991, Tracy Gordy, M.D., became the first psychiatrist to be appointed to the panel. He served as a member for 9 years and then as its chair for another 8 years until his retirement in November 2007.

The CPT Editorial Panel is supported by the CPT Advisory Committee, which has more than 90 members who represent all the specialty societies in the AMA's House of Delegates. The committee's main role is to advise the CPT Editorial Panel on the procedural coding and nomenclature that are relevant to each committee member's specialty. The committee also serves as a conduit through which revisions to CPT can be proposed by specialty societies or by individual members of those societies. (For more in-depth information on CPT, see Appendix A.)

The AMA's CPT coding system is now used universally throughout the United States. The Transactions Rule of the Health Insurance Portability and Accountability Act (HIPAA), which went into effect on October 16, 2002, required the use of CPT codes by all individuals and entities covered by HIPAA. (See Appendix B for basic information about HIPAA.) CPT codes constitute level I of the Healthcare Common Procedure Coding System used by Medicare and Medicaid. Every healthcare provider who receives payments from insurance companies needs to have a working knowledge of the CPT system. In truth, even those who do not receive payment from insurance companies need to be able to use the CPT system if their patients are to be able to file their own insurance claims for reimbursement.

CURRENT PROCEDURAL TERMINOLOGY MANUAL STRUCTURE

Physicians' Current Procedural Terminology (the CPT manual) is organized to be as user friendly as possible. The following is a quick survey of its contents.

Introduction

The short introduction contains valuable information for the clinician on how to use the manual, including

- a description and explanation of the format of the terminology (This section describes how some routine procedural terms are not repeated for subsequent related procedures to conserve entry space);
- a description of how to request updates of CPT (It is vital that physicians keep the AMA aware of changes in practice that require coding changes);
- a discussion of the specific guidelines that precede each of the manual's six sections (evaluation and management [E/M] and the five clinical sections);
- a discussion of "add-on codes" for additional or supplemental procedures;
- an explanation of code modifiers and how they are to be used;
- a brief discussion of how place of service relates to CPT;
- a discussion of the inclusion of codes for unlisted procedures or services in each section;
- a note that some CPT codes require interpretation and reporting if they are to be used;
- a note that special reports may be required to determine the medical appropriateness of rare or very new services;
- a discussion of how to identify code changes from year to year;
- a reference to the expanded alphabetical index now included in the manual;
- a note on how to obtain electronic versions of CPT; and finally
- how references to AMA resources on the CPT codes are noted in the manual.

Illustrated Anatomical and Procedural Review

This section provides a review of the basics of anatomy and medical vocabulary that are necessary for accurate coding. Lists of prefixes, suffixes, and roots are given, followed by 29 anatomical illustrations. There is also an index of all the procedural illustrations that appear throughout the manual, listed by their corresponding codes.

Evaluation and Management Codes

Although the rest of the CPT manual is organized according to the numerical order of the codes, the **evaluation and management (E/M) codes, 99201–99499,** are provided in the first code section because they are used by physicians in *all* specialties to report a considerable number of their services. The E/M codes are preceded by fairly extensive guidelines that define the terms used in the code descriptors and provide instructions for selecting the correct level of E/M service.

Major Clinical Sections

Next come the major clinical sections: Anesthesia, Surgery, Radiology, Pathology and Laboratory, and Medicine. Each of these sections is preceded by guidelines. **The psychiatry codes, 90801–90899, are found in the Medicine section.** The codes in the Psychiatry subsection cover most of the services mental health professionals provide to patients in both inpatient and outpatient settings.

Category II and III Codes

The Medicine section is followed by a listing of the supplemental Category II and Category III codes. These codes are generally optional codes used to facilitate data collection and are never used as a substitute for the Category I standard CPT codes.

Category II codes are used for performance measurement, such as the ongoing Physicians Quality Reporting Initiative currently being undertaken by Medicare. According to the CPT Manual, Category II codes are "intended to facilitate data collection about the quality of care rendered by coding certain services and test results that support nationally established performance measures and that have an evidence base as contributing to quality patient care."

Category III codes are temporary codes that are used to allow data tracking for emerging services and procedures.

Appendixes and Index

The last section of the CPT manual includes appendixes and an extensive alphabetical index. There are 13 appendixes:

- Appendix A: Modifiers—modifiers are two-digit suffixes that are added to CPT codes to indicate that the service or procedure has been provided under unusual circumstances (e.g., –21, which indicates a prolonged E/M service) (See Appendix C of this book for a list of modifiers.)
- Appendix B: Summary of Additions, Deletions, and Revisions (of codes in the current manual)
- Appendix C: Clinical Examples—provides clinical examples to clarify the use of E/M codes in various situations
- Appendix D: Summary of CPT Add-On Codes—codes used to denote procedures commonly carried out in addition to a primary procedure
- Appendix E: Summary of CPT Codes Exempt From Modifier –51 (multiple procedures)

- Appendix F: Summary of CPT Codes Exempt From Modifier –63 (which denotes a procedure perfomed on infants)
- Appendix G: Summary of CPT Codes That Include Moderate (Conscious) Sedation
- Appendix H: Alphabetic Index of Performance Measures by Clinical Condition or Topic (a listing of the diseases, clinical conditions, and topics with which the Category II codes are associated)
- Appendix I: Genetic Testing Code Modifiers (used "to provide diagnostic granularity of service to enable providers to submit complete and precise genetic testing information without altering test descriptors")
- Appendix J: Electrodiagnostic Medicine Listing of Sensory, Motor, and Mixed Nerves
- Appendix K: Products Pending FDA Approval (vaccine products that have been assigned a Category I code in anticipation of their approval by the U.S. Food and Drug Administration)
- Appendix L: Vascular Families
- Appendix M: Crosswalk to Deleted CPT Codes (indicating which current codes are to be used in place of the deleted ones)

The index is preceded by instructions explaining that there are four primary classes of index entries:

1. Procedure or Service
2. Organ or Other Anatomic Site
3. Condition
4. Synonyms, Eponyms, and Abbreviations

The instructions also explain the index's use of modifying terms, code ranges, and space-saving conventions.

QUESTIONS AND ANSWERS

Q. *How do I make suggestions about the introduction of new, or modifications for existing, CPT codes?*

A. If you are a psychiatrist, you can send your suggestions to the Office of Healthcare Systems and Financing at the American Psychiatric Association by e-mail to hsf@psych.org or by regular mail to 1000 Wilson Boulevard, Suite 1825, Arlington, VA 22209. Psychologists can send their suggestions to the American Psychological Association, 750 First Street, N.E., Washington, DC 20002. Psychiatric nurses can send their suggestions to the American Psychiatric Nurses Association at 1555 Wilson Boulevard, Suite 515, Arlington, VA 22209. Social workers can send their suggestions to the National Association of Social Workers, 750 First Street, N.E., Suite 700, Washington, DC 20002-4241. Suggestions can also be sent to the American Medical Association, CPT Research and Development, 515 North State Street, Chicago, IL 60654.

Q. *Do I really need to have an updated version of CPT every year?*

A. Yes, you need to have access to the most current edition of the CPT manual because there are additions and modifications every year.

Q. *Why don't insurance companies pay for all the procedures listed in CPT?*

A. CPT is a coding system only. Insurance companies must use this system for recording procedures, but they are not obligated to pay for every procedure listed in the coding system.

Q. *If I'm unsure how to code for a service I've provided, what can I do?*

A. The American Psychiatric Association provides a coding service for its members through its Office of Healthcare Systems and Financing. The AMA and other specialty associations may provide this service as well. See Appendix L for more information.

2

Introduction to Documentation of Psychiatric Services

Accurate, understandable documentation is essential for providing ongoing patient care for the following reasons:

1. Accurate documentation is good medicine. Clear, concise recording of the when, what, and why of the services you provide to patients is an intrinsic component of good care. Documentation also clarifies the medical necessity that guides the reasoning on which treatment planning is based and contributes to continuity of care by facilitating communication between the various health professionals who are involved in the patient's care.

2. Accurate documentation is the basis for selecting both procedural and diagnostic codes. It is the way medical necessity is expressed. Your diagnosis (diagnoses) of the patient's condition(s) (noted using the DSM/ICD diagnostic codes) is dependent on the content of the initial evaluation (history, examination, laboratory tests). What you did for the patient as documented in the medical record is matched to the descriptors of the Current Procedural Terminology (CPT) codes, allowing you to select the most appropriate code. Both the diagnostic and the procedure codes are essential for payment and claims review.

3. Accurate documentation is your best protection against audit liability. First, documentation assists in accurate coding, which reduces the chances of an audit. Second, if you are audited, documentation provides the factual database that supports your coding and charges.

4. Accurate documentation protects you if you are accused of malpractice. Your records will support your rationale for having made medical decisions and will demonstrate what, in fact, you did for the patient.

As the requirement for evidence-based medicine becomes more and more pervasive, it is vital that the documentation in the patient's medical record make clear the medical necessity for the course of care provided. For mental health services, many payers use a resource for making their payment decisions about medical necessity and level of care called the InterQual Behavioral Health Criteria, published by McKesson Health Solutions, LLC. The InterQual criteria comprise six manuals covering psychiatry: adult (patients 17–65 years old); geriatric (age 65 and older); child (ages 4–12 years); adolescent (ages 13–17 years); residential treatment; and chemical dependency and dual diagnosis. Each manual has more than 200 pages and presents a review process that uses algorithms and criteria sets that were developed by physicians and other healthcare professionals. McKesson states that the clinical content of its manuals "is a synthesis of evidence based standards of care, current practices, and consensus from licensed specialists and/or primary care physicians." Although most practicing clinicians have probably never even seen the manuals published by McKesson (not just for behavioral health but for all of medicine), they have a profound effect on healthcare reimbursements in the United States.

Another benefit of taking coding and documentation seriously is that more and more physician reimbursement models for commercial and public payers are being based on "risk adjustment" of the patient population that is being served. Examples of risk-adjusted reimbursement models include capitation, global payment, and the patient-centered medical home. Risk adjustment methodology is based on claims data, which include diagnoses, patient demographics, and the use of medical services to place patients in low, medium, or high levels of morbidity relative to the total population in the patient's health plan.

Numerous studies of risk-adjusted patient populations have demonstrated that although patients with a high morbidity rating account for only 7%–10% of a given health plan's membership, they are responsible for 75%–80% of the plan's health costs. This reality has caused providers and payers to target the high morbidity segment of the patient population for preventive services, case management, and chronic disease management—all of which have been shown to reduce the cost of medical care for these patients.

In recognition of the increased physician work associated with these extra services, reimbursement is often increased for caring for patients with high morbidity (**more diagnoses = higher morbidity = more work = higher reimbursement**). Using CPT coding and documentation and the DSM-IV-TR Multiaxial Assessment is a near perfect method for making explicit the level of morbidity of any psychiatric patient.

The CPT code denotes the type and intensity of physician work. Documentation supports the selection of the code by making explicit the extent of the work involved in taking the history and doing the examination within the context of the complexity of medical decision making. The Multiaxial Assessment is a concise means of diagnostically presenting psychiatric/medical complexity and functional status.

Using these tools puts psychiatrists and other mental health professionals in an excellent position to be able to actively participate in new reimbursement models that are based on risk adjustment methodologies.

DOCUMENTATION PRINCIPLES

The following documentation principles are based on those published in 1992 by the American Medical Association (AMA):

- The medical record should be **complete** and **legible.**
- The documentation of each patient encounter should include

  - the date;
  - the reason for the encounter;
  - the appropriate history and results of a physical examination;
  - a review of laboratory findings, X-ray data, and other ancillary services, if appropriate;
  - an assessment; and
  - a plan for care, including a discharge plan, if appropriate.

- The reasons for and results of X-rays, laboratory tests, and other ancillary services should be documented or included in the medical record.
- Past and present diagnoses should be accessible to the treating and/or consulting physician.
- Relevant health risk factors should be identified.
- The patient's progress should be documented, including

  - response to treatment;
  - change in treatment plan;
  - change in diagnosis; and
  - any nonadherence with treatment.

- The treatment plan should include, when appropriate

  - treatments and medications, specifying frequency and dosage;
  - any referrals and consultations;
  - patient/family education; and
  - specific instructions for follow-up.

- The documentation should support the intensity of the patient's evaluation and/or treatment by including a record of the treating physician's thought processes and the complexity of medical decision making.
- All entries to the medical record should be **dated** and **authenticated (signed).**
- The content of the medical report supports the selection of the **DSM/ICD diagnostic code** and the **CPT service code.**

These general principles can be used for handwritten notes, dictated notes, filling out preprinted template forms, or completing templates embedded in electronic patient records. Regardless of the method of production, clinical notes that contain the information included in the AMA documentation principles will meet the requirements of all commercial payers and Medicare. Because Medicare generally has the most stringent documentation requirements, these specific requirements are the ones provided throughout this handbook.

Documentation of psychiatric evaluation and therapeutic procedures (the 908xx series) is discussed in Chapter 3. Documentation for evaluation and management procedures (the 99xxx series) is discussed in Chapter 4.

Documentation for the psychiatric service codes has been complicated by Health Insurance Portability and Accountability Act (HIPAA) requirements that create a more stringent level of privacy protection for psychotherapy notes (those personal notes that do not contain information that would be defined as part of the medical record) than for the rest of the patient's medical record as long as those notes can be physically separated from the rest of the record. In fact, if documentation has been done correctly, it will not include any information that is considered "psychotherapy notes." (For more information about HIPAA and the definition of psychotherapy notes, see Appendix B.)

The reality is that providers must meet community standards of documentation for the clinical needs of their patients and at the same time must meet the administrative documentation requirements of insurers in order to be appropriately reimbursed and remain in compliance with regulatory and institutional requirements. Complying with these two sets of requirements must be done efficiently because record creation (i.e., documentation) is already accounted for in the relative value units of both the evaluation and management and psychiatry codes as pre- and postservice work. Translated, this means that although thorough medical record keeping is essential for good patient care as well as for reimbursement, and can be very time-consuming, the time it takes to create the medical record is not directly reimbursed. Consequently, it is best to find a way to document that allows you to do it as efficiently as possible, such as using templates. Appendix H provides examples of preprinted documentation templates.

3

Codes and Documentation for Psychiatric Services and Other Mental Health Services

Psychiatric evaluation and therapeutic procedure codes are a subsection of the CPT manual's Medicine section (pp. 429–500 in the *2010 CPT Manual, Professional Edition*). These codes are the "bread and butter" codes for psychiatrists, psychologists, social workers, and other mental health professionals. They are used to denote the services clinicians provide to patients in a variety of clinical settings (see Chapter 5 for a discussion of coding in these settings).

The introductory notes to the Psychiatry subsection provide vital information about the codes and how they are to be used. For example, the notes instruct the reader on the use of evaluation and management (E/M) codes for attending hospital care, the combined use of E/M hospital care codes and psychiatric therapeutic procedure codes, which psychiatric therapeutic codes cannot be used with E/M codes, and under what conditions E/M consultation codes should be used (see Chapter 4 for a discussion of E/M codes). The notes also briefly describe the use of modifiers; for example, –22 for a service that is more extensive than usual and –52 for a service that is reduced or less extensive than usual. The answers to many of the coding questions that are handled by the American Psychiatric Association's CPT Coding Service can be found in these introductory notes.

As of this printing, there are no agreed-on, nationally accepted documentation standards for the 908xx series of codes. The documentation elements presented for the codes that follow have been created based on a survey of documentation requirements published by Medicare contractors across the nation. You will note that in the main these documentation elements closely match many of the elements of the American Medical Association's (AMA's) documentation principles discussed in Chapter 2.

PSYCHIATRIC DIAGNOSTIC OR EVALUATIVE INTERVIEW PROCEDURES

90801   **CPT descriptor:** Psychiatric diagnostic interview examination

Code 90801 is used for an *initial* diagnostic interview examination and may be used in both outpatient and inpatient settings. Psychiatrists use the E/M codes for initial hospital care (99221–99223) more frequently than 90801 when doing an initial evaluation in an inpatient setting, and E/M codes may be used for outpatient care as well (see Chapter 4 for information on E/M codes). 90801 is also appropriate to use for consultations in both inpatient and outpatient settings now that Medicare no longer pays for consultation codes.

The elements of 90801 include

- Identification of a chief complaint
- History of present illness
- Past medical history
- Past psychiatric history
- Family and social history
- Complete mental status examination
- Diagnosis
- Ordering and medical interpretation of laboratory or other diagnostic studies
- Treatment plan and disposition

Payment Policy Issues.   Most insurers, including Medicare, will pay for a 90801 if it is necessitated by a new episode. Medicare will pay for only one evaluation per year for an institutionalized patient (psychiatric hospital or nursing home) unless medical necessity can be established for additional evaluations (a change in mental status, the development of a new psychiatric condition).

Medicare allows physicians to use either 90801 or the appropriate inpatient E/M code (99221–99223) for the diagnostic interview on the first day of hospitalization. If the highest level of E/M is appropriate, using 99223 instead of 90801 may result in higher reimbursement for the evaluation. One of the differences between the two codes is that the 99223 *requires that a complete review of systems be done and documented.* The review of systems may be done by the attending psychiatrist or by the physician who completes the medical history and physical examination. In the latter instance, the attending psychiatrist must review and countersign the review of systems done by the other physician and comment on pertinent positives and negatives.

> **Warning:** Psychiatrists who use the 99223 code instead of 90801 frequently encounter payment problems because of a failure to completely document the review of systems.

It is important to note that codes 90801 and 90802, which is used for interactive psychiatric diagnostic interviews, are not subject to the outpatient mental health services limitation under Medicare (see Chapter 6). These two codes have always been reimbursed at 80% like all other medical codes rather than at the 50% rate that had been used for other outpatient psychiatric codes. This payment anomaly is being phased out gradually, and in 2010 outpatient psychiatric treatment codes are being reimbursed at 55%. In 2014 all psychiatric services will be paid at 80%.

Although 90801 is not a timed code, the community standard for 90801 is between 45 minutes and 1 hour. For instances in which the evaluation takes longer, the CPT modifier −22, "unusual procedural services," should be used (see Appendix C for a list of modifiers). Be sure to document the extra time and explain why it was required. Child and geriatric psychiatrists often require more than one session to complete a psychiatric evaluation. It is recommended that when more than one session is necessary the psychiatrist check with the patient's insurer to determine how to code for appropriate reimbursement.

Documentation.   It is recommended that documentation for 90801 include the following elements:

- Date
- Chief complaint
- Referral source
- History of present illness
- Past psychiatric history
- Past medical history
- Social and family history
- Comprehensive mental status examination
- Formulation/prognosis
- Treatment plan
- Assessment of the patient's ability to adhere to the treatment plan
- Multiaxial diagnoses
- Signature (if not legible, must include printed name)

See the template for Attending Consultant Physician Psychiatry Evaluation in Appendix H. Note that the review of systems on the template is not necessary for 90801.

90802   **CPT descriptor:** Interactive psychiatric diagnostic interview examination using play equipment, physical devices, language interpreter, or other mechanisms of communication

Code 90802 was designed to be used primarily for the evaluation of young children, but it may also be used for the evaluation of adults who have impaired cognitive or communication abilities. To be interactive, the evaluation must include the use of physical aids or nonverbal communication to overcome barriers to therapeutic interaction between the psychiatrist and the patient. When an interpreter is used for sign language or any other language, 90802 is the appropriate code.

Payment Policy Issues.   Services designated with this code are covered by most insurance plans, but medical necessity for using the interactive code must be documented.

Documentation. Documentation is the same as for 90801, with the additional requirement that the interactive devices employed should be described, as should the condition that necessitated their use.

PSYCHIATRIC THERAPEUTIC PROCEDURES

The CPT manual section for Psychiatric Therapeutic Procedures divides the basic psychotherapy codes, 90804–90829 (delineated as being for insight-oriented, behavior-modifying, and/or supportive psychotherapy and those for interactive psychotherapy) by the setting in which they occur: outpatient or inpatient. It then has a section for "Other Psychotherapy," codes 90845–90857, which includes psychoanalysis and various types of family and group psychotherapy. The final section in the Psychiatry section is for "Other Psychiatric Services or Procedures," codes 90862–90899, which covers a broad spectrum of services, from the frequently used pharmacological management to hypnotherapy and preparation of a psychiatric status report.

The Psychotherapy Codes

The psychotherapy codes distinguish between psychotherapy provided **with evaluation and management (E/M) services** and **without E/M services**. The E/M services provided with psychotherapy may include but are not limited to

- medication management;
- medical diagnostic evaluations (e.g., evaluation of comorbid medical conditions, drug interactions);
- writing physician orders;
- checking lithium levels; and
- taking blood pressure.

Only physicians and duly licensed physician assistants and nurse practitioners may use the codes for psychotherapy with E/M services. Codes for psychotherapy with E/M services are reimbursed at a slightly higher rate than for psychotherapy without E/M, even though the codes designate that they take the same amount of time, because the total work of psychotherapy with E/M is deemed greater (approximately 2–5 minutes of practitioner work could be said to account for the higher rate, or 0.16 relative value units).

The appropriate code for psychotherapy is selected on the basis of

- Time spent face-to-face with the patient;
- The kind of therapy that is provided (insight-oriented, behavior-modifying, and/or supportive psychotherapy);
- Whether E/M services are provided;
- Whether the service is interactive; and
- Whether the service occurs in an outpatient or inpatient setting.

CODES FOR PSYCHOTHERAPY IN AN OFFICE OR OTHER OUTPATIENT FACILITY

CPT descriptor: Insight-oriented, behavior-modifying, and/or supportive psychotherapy

> **Note:** This list of psychotherapy modes is not meant to be exclusive, but rather is representational, and therapy modes such as cognitive-behavioral therapy would also be included in the codes that bear this descriptor.

90804	20–30 minutes
90805	20–30 minutes with E/M
90806	45–50 minutes
90807	45–50 minutes with E/M
90808	75–80 minutes
90809	75–80 minutes with E/M

CPT descriptor: Interactive psychotherapy

90810	20–30 minutes
90811	20–30 minutes with E/M
90812	45–50 minutes
90813	45–50 minutes with E/M
90814	75–80 minutes
90815	75–80 minutes with E/M

> **Warning:** The clinician should be cautious about using the interactive psychotherapy codes and carefully follow the instructions provided by the CPT manual if these codes are used. The codes for interactive psychotherapy are primarily used for services provided to children or to adults who can benefit from psychotherapy but do not have the capacity to communicate verbally.

Documentation. There are no universally accepted standard guidelines for psychotherapy services similar to the documentation guidelines for E/M services. Many Medicare contractors publish documentation requirements as part of their Local Coverage Determination policies for the psychotherapy codes, but these requirements vary from contractor to contractor. If you include the following information in your documentation of psychotherapy, you should meet the requirements for both Medicare and commercial payers:

- Date of service
- Time spent for the encounter face-to-face
- Type of therapeutic intervention (i.e., insight oriented, supportive, behavior modification)
- Target symptoms
- Progress toward achievement of treatment goals
- E/M services provided (e.g., medication management or assessment of patient's physical health), if service provided is psychotherapy with E/M

- Diagnoses
- If therapy is interactive, reason interactive therapy is required and method used for the interaction
- For 90814 and 90815 and other codes for more than 50 minutes of therapy, explanation as to why session required this length of time
- Legible signature

CODES FOR PSYCHOTHERAPY IN AN INPATIENT HOSPITAL, PARTIAL HOSPITAL, OR RESIDENTIAL CARE FACILITY

CPT descriptor: Insight-oriented, behavior-modifying, and/or supportive psychotherapy

90816	20–30 minutes
90817	20–30 minutes with E/M
90818	45–50 minutes
90819	45–50 minutes with E/M
90821	75–80 minutes
90822	75–80 minutes with E/M

CPT descriptor: Interactive psychotherapy

90823	20–30 minutes
90824	20–30 minutes with E/M
90826	45–50 minutes
90827	45–50 minutes with E/M
90828	75–80 minutes
90829	75–80 minutes with E/M

> **Warning:** The clinician should be cautious about using the interactive psychotherapy codes and carefully follow the instructions provided by the CPT manual if these codes are used. The codes for interactive psychotherapy are primarily used for services provided to children or adults who can benefit from psychotherapy but do not have the capacity to communicate verbally.

Documentation.   Documentation is the same as for other psychotherapy services. See notes on documentation for psychotherapy in an office or other outpatient facility.

Other Psychotherapy Codes

90845   **CPT descriptor:** Psychoanalysis

Psychoanalysis is performed by therapists who are trained and credentialed to practice psychoanalysis. Psychoanalysis is reported on a per-session basis, and most insurance programs will provide reimbursement for this service. Note that although 90845 does not prescribe time, psychoanalytic sessions are usually considered to be 50 minutes long.

> **Warning:** Because of the frequency of sessions, the issue of medical necessity has resulted in challenges to reimbursement for psychoanalysis by many managed care companies.

Documentation. Documentation is the same as for other psychotherapy services. See "Codes for Psychotherapy in an Office or Other Outpatient Facility." Although this is not a timed code, payers will expect time spent to meet community standards.

90846   **CPT descriptor:** Family psychotherapy (without the patient present)

Code 90846 is used when the clinician provides therapy for the family of a patient without the patient being present. Under Medicare rules, procedures designated with code 90846 are covered only if the therapy is clearly directed toward the treatment of the patient, rather than toward helping family members who may have issues because of the patient's illness. A session of family psychotherapy (without the patient present) typically lasts 45 minutes to 1 hour.

Payment Policy Issues. Although most insurance companies will reimburse for services designated with this code, problems may occur because the service is not face-to-face with the patient. This issue is of particular concern to clinicians who treat children/adolescents and geriatric patients. They frequently must spend evaluation, treatment, and education time with parents, children, or other caregivers without the patient being present. Most payers have been alerted to this problem, and some have unofficially suggested that clinicians use 90847 (see the discussion of code 90847 later in this section) as long as the patient is physically present for some portion of the session.

Documentation. Documentation is the same as for other psychotherapy services (see "Codes for Psychotherapy in an Office or Other Outpatient Facility"), with the addition of a list of family members present during the session. Although this is not a timed code, payers will expect time spent to meet community standards.

> **Warning:** In documenting services coded 90846 for reimbursement by Medicare, it is essential to state that the service was provided for the treatment of the covered patient, not for the family members who were present.

90847   **CPT descriptor:** Family psychotherapy (conjoint psychotherapy) (with patient present)

Code 90847 is used when the therapy includes the patient and family members. Code 90847 should also be used for couples therapy. A session of family psychotherapy (conjoint psychotherapy) (with the patient present) typically lasts 45 minutes to 1 hour.

Payment Policy Issues. Services designated with this code are covered by most insurance plans and, because the patient is present, are challenged less frequently than those coded 90846.

Documentation. Documentation is the same as for other psychotherapy services (see "Codes for Psychotherapy in an Office or Other Outpatient Facility"), with the addition of a list of those present during the session. Although this is not a timed code, payers will expect time spent to meet community standards.

90849   **CPT descriptor:** Multiple-family group psychotherapy

Code 90849 is used when the clinician provides psychotherapy to a group of adult or adolescent patients and their family members. The usual treatment strategy is to modify family behavior and attitudes. The service is covered by most insurance plans. Group psychotherapy sessions are typically 1 hour long.

Documentation. Documentation is the same as for other psychotherapy services (see "Codes for Psychotherapy in an Office or Other Outpatient Facility"), with the addition of a list of the family members present. **Documentation of the service must be provided for each patient's record.** Although this is not a timed code, payers will expect time spent to meet community standards.

90853   **CPT descriptor:** Group psychotherapy (other than of a multiple-family group)

Services that are coded 90853 rely on the use of interactions of group members to examine the pathology of each individual within the group. In addition, the dynamics of the entire group are noted and used to modify behaviors and attitudes of the patient members. The size of the group may vary depending on the therapeutic goals of the group and/or the type of therapeutic interactions used by the therapist. The code is used to report per-session services for each group member. The typical time for a group psychotherapy session is 1 hour, and most insurance plans cover this treatment.

Documentation. Documentation is the same as for other psychotherapy services. See notes on documentation for psychotherapy in an office or other outpatient facility. Although this is not a timed code, payers will expect time spent to meet community standards. **Individual documentation must be provided for each group member's record.**

90857   **CPT descriptor:** Interactive group psychotherapy

Code 90857 is used when clinicians provide psychotherapy using nonverbal communication and activities, such as play therapy, with young children in groups. Similar procedures might be necessary for adult patients who have impaired communication skills. Typical time for a session is 1 hour.

> **Warning:** This code should not be used for adults unless medical necessity can be and is documented. All insurance carriers, including Medicare, will audit psychiatrists who routinely use this procedure for adults.

Documentation. Documentation is the same as for group psychotherapy, with the addition of documentation of the interactive tools that were used as well as the reasons for using interactive therapy. **Documentation must be provided for each group member.**

OTHER PSYCHIATRIC SERVICES OR PROCEDURES

90862   **CPT descriptor:** Pharmacological management, including prescription use, and review of medication, with no more than minimal medical psychotherapy

Because 90862 is used so frequently by psychiatrists, it is closely monitored by the Medicare program. Although 90862 is not a time-delineated code, within the Medicare program the expectation is that the work represents at least 15 minutes face-to-face with the patient.

Prescription refills or medication management that takes less than 15 minutes should be coded with an E/M office visit code, level 2—99212 for an established patient, with an average time of 10 minutes, or for Medicare patients the M0064 code should be used (see table). It also represents 10 minutes of work.

Code	Average time, *minutes*	Non-facility fee
99212 Office/outpatient visit, established	10	$38.97
M0064 Visit for drug monitoring	10	$42.22
90862 Medication management	15 or more	$56.29

Note.   Fees are approximate.

If psychotherapy is provided at all, it should be brief and supportive.

Under the Medicare program, when 90862 is provided for a patient with the diagnosis of Alzheimer's disease or an Alzheimer's-like dementia, it is exempt from the current outpatient mental health services limitation and is reimbursed at 80% (see information about the fate of the limitation under 90801).

Documentation.   Documentation should include

- the date;
- time spent face-to-face with the patient;
- interval history;
- diagnosis;
- relevant mental status examination results;
- response to medications;
- review of side effects;
- prescription provided;
- any relevant laboratory monitoring (i.e., lithium level); and
- a legible signature.

See Appendix H for a template containing these elements.

90865   **CPT descriptor:** Narcosynthesis for psychiatric diagnostic and therapeutic purposes (e.g., sodium amobarbital [Amytal] interview)

This procedure involves the administration, usually through slow intravenous infusion, of a barbiturate or a benzodiazepine in order to suppress inhibitions, allowing the patient to reveal and discuss material that could not be verbalized without the disinhibiting effect of the medication.

Documentation.   Documentation should include date, diagnosis, target symptoms, and signature as well as a description of the procedure, the medications used, the patient's response to the procedure, and a brief account of the material verbalized under narcosynthesis and whether treatment goals were achieved.

90870   **CPT descriptor:** Electroconvulsive therapy (includes necessary monitoring)

This code includes the time the psychiatrist takes to monitor the patient during the preparation, convulsive phase, and recovery phase of electroconvulsive therapy (ECT). When the psychiatrist also administers the anesthesia, the anesthesia service should be coded and reported separately.

Documentation.   See Appendix I for ECT documentation record.

90875   **CPT descriptor:** Individual psychophysiological therapy
and   incorporating biofeedback training by any modality (face-to-face
90876   with the patient) with psychotherapy (e.g., insight-oriented, behavior-modifying, and/or supportive psychotherapy)
90875: approximately 20–30 minutes
90876: approximately 45–50 minutes

These two procedures incorporate biofeedback and psychotherapy (insight oriented, behavior modifying, and/or supportive) as combined modalities conducted face-to-face with the patient. They are distinct from biofeedback codes 90901 and 90911, which do not incorporate psychotherapy and do not require face-to-face time.

Payment Policy Issues.   Medicare will not reimburse for services designated with codes 90901 and 90911.

Documentation.   Documentation should include date, diagnosis, target symptoms, and signature plus a description of the procedure and its outcome.

90880   **CPT descriptor:** Hypnotherapy

Hypnosis is the procedure of inducing a passive state in which the patient demonstrates increased amenability and responsiveness to suggestions and commands, provided they do not conflict seriously with the patient's conscious or unconscious wishes. Hypnotherapy may be used for either diagnostic or treatment purposes.

Documentation.   Documentation should include the standard information stipulated for the psychotherapy codes plus a description of the procedure and its outcome.

90882   **CPT descriptor:** Environmental intervention for medical management purposes on a psychiatric patient's behalf with agencies, employers, or institutions

The activities covered by code 90882 include visits by a clinician to the patient's worksite to improve work conditions for the patient, visits to community-based organizations on behalf of a chronically mentally ill patient to discuss a change in living conditions, and accompanying a patient with a phobia in order to help desensitize the patient to a stimulus. Other activities include coordination of services with agencies, employers, or institutions.

Payment Policy Issues.   This service is covered by some insurance plans, but because some of the activities are not face-to-face with the patient, the clinician should check with carriers about their willingness to reimburse for services designated with this code. Medicare does not pay for services designated with this code, which means that as long as the patient is informed in advance that fees for this service will have to be paid for out of pocket, the clinician is free to charge Medicare patients the same fee that private patients are charged. Clinicians are advised to have the patient acknowledge in writing that he or she understands that this service is not covered and to keep a copy of the acknowledgment in the patient's file.

Documentation.   Documentation should include date, time, and signature, plus a description of the actions performed on the patient's behalf.

90885   **CPT descriptor:** Psychiatric evaluation of hospital records, other psychiatric reports, psychometric and/or projective tests, and other accumulated data for medical diagnostic purposes

Payment Policy Issues.   Code 90885 would seem to denote a very useful activity, but because reviewing data is not a face-to-face service with the patient, Medicare will not reimburse for it, and some commercial health insurance carriers have followed suit. Medicare considers the review of data to be part of the pre- and postwork associated with any face-to-face service.

Documentation.   Documentation should include date, time, and signature, plus an account of which records were reviewed.

90887   **CPT descriptor:** Interpretation or explanation of results of psychiatric, other medical examinations and procedures, or other accumulated data to family or other responsible persons, or advising them how to assist patient

Payment Policy Issues.   Medicare will not reimburse for this service because it is not done face-to-face with the patient, and clinicians should verify coverage by other insurers to ensure reimbursement. It is appropriate to use an E/M code for this service in the hospital, where floor time is expressed as coordination of care with the time documented. As with other services that are not covered by Medicare, if the patient still wishes this service to be provided after being informed that Medicare will not reimburse for it, the clinician is free to charge his or her established office fee. Clinicians are advised to have the patient acknowledge in writing that he or she understands that this service is not covered and to keep a copy of the acknowledgment in the patient's file.

Documentation. Documentation should include date, time, and signature as well as an account of the material reviewed.

90889   **CPT descriptor:** Preparation of report of patient's psychiatric status, history, treatment, or progress (other than for legal or consultative purposes) for other physicians, agencies, or insurance carriers

Psychiatrists are often called on to prepare reports about a patient for other participants in the health care system. Code 90889 would be best used to denote this service. However, because this service is not provided face-to-face with the patient, Medicare will not reimburse for services designated with this code, and clinicians should verify coverage by other insurers. Again, if a Medicare patient still wishes the clinician to prepare such a report, the patient may be asked to pay the practitioner's standard fee out of pocket. As with other noncovered services, the clinician should have the patient acknowledge in writing that he or she understands the service is not covered, and the acknowledgment should be kept in the patient's file.

Documentation. A copy of the report, including date, time, and signature, is the appropriate documentation for this code.

90899   **CPT descriptor:** Unlisted psychiatric service or procedure

Code 90899 is used for services not specifically defined under any other code. It might also be used for procedures that require some degree of explanation or justification. If the code is used under these circumstances, a brief, jargon-free note explaining the use of the code to the insurance carrier is often helpful in obtaining reimbursement. If the code is used for a service that is not provided face-to-face with a patient, the psychiatrist should check with the patient's insurer regarding reimbursement.

Documentation. Documentation for this code should include date, time, and signature as well as a legible explanation of the service or procedure provided and why it was medically necessary.

M0064   **Descriptor:** Brief office visit for the sole purpose of monitoring or changing drug prescriptions used in the treatment of mental, psychoneurotic, and personality disorders

M0064 is not, in fact, a CPT code. It is a level II code within the Healthcare Common Procedure Coding System used by Medicare and Medicaid (CPT codes are level I). M0064 should be used only for the briefest medication check with stable patients in an office setting (see 90862 earlier in the chapter for more information).

Documentation. Documentation should include the usual identifying information (place, time, signature) as well as the name of the medication being checked and reasons for continuation or changes in medication.

NONPSYCHIATRIC MENTAL HEALTH SERVICES

Besides the CPT psychiatry codes discussed earlier in the chapter (the 908xx series), a number of other codes are used by mental health professionals. These codes are also found in the Medicine section of the CPT manual. We present them here in the order in which they appear in the manual.

Sleep Testing

These codes are listed as a subsection of the Neurology and Neuromuscular Procedures codes. The sleep testing codes are premised on studies of 6 hours or more, and a –52 modifier is to be used if the procedure lasts for less time.

95805   **CPT descriptor:** Sleep latency or maintenance of wakefulness testing, recording, analysis, and interpretation of physiological measurements of sleep during multiple trials to assess sleepiness

Documentation. A report that includes the study results is the appropriate documentation for this code.

95806   **CPT descriptor:** Sleep study, simultaneous recording of ventilation, respiratory effort, electrocardiogram or heart rate, and oxygen saturation, unattended by a technologist

Documentation. A report that includes the study results is the appropriate documentation for this code.

95807   **CPT descriptor:** Sleep study, simultaneous recording of ventilation, respiratory effort, electrocardiogram or heart rate, and oxygen saturation, attended by a technologist

Documentation. A report that includes the study results is the appropriate documentation for this code.

95808   **CPT descriptor:** Polysomnography; sleep staging with one to three additional parameters of sleep, attended by a technologist

Documentation.   A report that includes the study results is the appropriate documentation for this code.

95810   **CPT descriptor:** …sleep staging with four or more additional parameters of sleep, attended by a technologist

Documentation.   Documentation is the same as for sleep staging with one to four or more additional parameters, with the additional parameters documented.

95811   **CPT descriptor:** …sleep staging with four or more additional parameters of sleep, with initiation of continuous positive airway pressure therapy or bilevel ventilation, attended by a technologist

Documentation.   Documentation is the same as for sleep staging with four or more additional parameters, with the additional information documented.

Central Nervous System Assessments/Tests

These codes are used to report services provided as part of the testing of the cognitive function of the central nervous system, including neurocognitive, mental status, and speech testing. It is expected that a combination of testing procedures will be used. It is also expected that this testing will generate material that will be used to write a report. The report created serves as the documentation for these services.

96101   **CPT descriptor:** Psychological testing (includes psychodiagnostic assessment of emotionality, intellectual abilities, personality, and psychopathology, e.g., Minnesota Multiphasic Personality Inventory, Rorschach, Wechsler Adult Intelligence Scale), per hour of the psychologist's or physician's time, both face-to-face time administering tests to the patient and time interpreting these test results and preparing the report

Documentation.   The report serves as the documentation for this code.

96102   **CPT descriptor:** Psychological testing (includes psychodiagnostic assessment of emotionality, intellectual abilities, personality and psychopathology, e.g., Minnesota Multiphasic Personality Inventory and Wechsler Adult Intelligence Scale), with qualified healthcare professional interpretation and report, administered by technician, per hour of technician time, face-to-face

Documentation.   The report serves as the documentation for this code.

96103   **CPT descriptor:** Psychological testing (includes psychodiagnostic assessment of emotionality, intellectual abilities, personality and psychopathology, e.g., Minnesota Multiphasic Personality Inventory), administered by computer, with qualified healthcare professional interpretation and report

Documentation.   The report serves as the documentation for this code.

96105   **CPT descriptor:** Assessment of aphasia (includes assessment of expressive and receptive speech and language function, language comprehension, speech production ability, reading, spelling, and writing, e.g., by Boston Diagnostic Aphasia Examination) with interpretation and report, per hour

Documentation.   The report serves as the documentation for this code.

96110 and 96111   **96110 CPT descriptor:** Developmental testing; limited (e.g., Developmental Screening Test II, Early Language Milestone Screen) with interpretation and report

96111 CPT descriptor: Developmental testing; extended (includes assessment of motor, language, social, adaptive, and/or cognitive functioning by standardized development instruments) with interpretation and report

Documentation.   The report serves as the documentation for both of these codes.

96116   **CPT descriptor:** Neurobehavioral status examination (clinical assessment of thinking, reasoning, and judgment, e.g., acquired knowledge; attention, language, memory, planning and problem solving; and visual-spatial abilities) per hour of the psychologist's or physician's time, both face-to-face time with the patient and time interpreting test results and preparing the report

Documentation.   The report serves as the documentation for this code.

96118   **CPT descriptor:** Neuropsychological testing (e.g., Halstead-Reitan Neuropsychological Battery, Wechsler Memory Scales, and Wisconsin Card Sorting Test) per hour of the psychologist's or physician's time, both face-to-face time administering tests to the patient and time interpreting these test results and preparing the report

Documentation.   The report serves as the documentation for this code.

96119   **CPT descriptor:** Neuropsychological testing (e.g., Halstead-Reitan Neuropsychological Battery, Wechsler Memory Scales, and Wisconsin Card Sorting Test), with qualified healthcare professional interpretation and report, administered by technician, per hour of technician time, face-to-face

Documentation.   The report serves as the documentation for this code.

96120   **CPT descriptor:** Neuropsychological testing (e.g., Wisconsin Card Sorting Test) administered by a computer, with qualified healthcare professional interpretation and report

Documentation.   The report serves as the documentation for this code.

96125   **CPT descriptor:** Standardized cognitive performance testing (e.g., Ross Information Processing Assessment) per hour of a qualified healthcare professional's time, both face-to-face time administering the tests to the patient and time interpreting these test results and preparing the report

Documentation.   The report serves as the documentation for this code.

Health and Behavior Assessment/Intervention

These codes were specifically created to be used for determining the psychological, behavioral, emotional, cognitive, and social factors that affect the patient's physical health. It is important that you read the narrative introduction to these codes in the CPT manual to be sure you understand how they are to be used. The focus is not on mental health but rather on the biopsychosocial factors that have bearing on the patient's physical health. The idea is to improve the patient's physical health by using cognitive, behavioral, social, and/ or psychophysiological procedures that will ameliorate disease-related problems. These codes denote services associated with an acute or a chronic illness (not psychiatric in nature), prevention of a physical illness, and maintenance of health. They do not represent preventive medicine services. The patients who receive these services have not received a diagnosis of a mental illness but have a physical illness or symptoms, and it is believed that the treatment of the condition may benefit from a focus on psychosocial issues. If a patient requires both a health and behavior assessment/intervention and a psychiatric service, only the most predominant service should be recorded. The codes cannot be used for services provided on the same day the patient is provided with a psychiatric service. Physicians performing health and behavioral assessments or interventions should use the appropriate E/M or preventive medicine service codes.

**96150
and
96151**

96150 CPT descriptor: Health and behavior assessment (e.g., health-focused clinical interview, behavioral observations, psychophysiological monitoring, health-oriented questionnaires), each 15 minutes face-to-face with the patient; initial assessment

96151 CPT descriptor: …reassessment

Documentation. The documentation for these codes consists of a report of the evaluation methods used, observations, results of psychophysiological monitoring, a summary of the assessment, recommendations, the number of 15-minute units, and the total time spent with the patient.

**96152–
96155**

96152 CPT descriptor: Health and behavior intervention, each 15 minutes face-to-face; individual

96153 CPT descriptor: …group (two or more patients)

96154 CPT descriptor: …family (with the patient present)

96155 CPT descriptor: …family (without the patient present)

Documentation. The documentation for these codes consists of a report of the intervention methods used, observations, results of psychophysiological monitoring, a summary of the intervention, any recommendations arising from the intervention, the number of 15-minute units, and the total time spent with the patient or family.

QUESTIONS AND ANSWERS

Q. *Who can provide psychiatric diagnostic or evaluative interview procedures (codes 90801 and 90802)?*

A. All mental health professionals who are licensed in their states to perform these services, including psychiatrists, clinical psychologists, certified clinical social workers, psychiatric nurse-practitioners, clinical nurse specialists, and physician assistants.

Q. *How do I choose between a psychotherapy code with E/M and code 90862?*

A. Look to the primary service you provided. If you have seen the patient just for medication management and provided no or only minimal psychotherapy, choose 90862. If you have primarily had a psychotherapy session during which you briefly evaluated the patient's medication regimen, choose the appropriate psychotherapy code with E/M.

Q. *If two professionals in a group practice are required to do independent evaluations of a patient within days of each other, can they both use code 90801?*

A. Yes, but payment will depend on the policy of the insurer, so check first.

Q. *If I provide a unique psychotherapeutic service on a recurrent basis, do I have to use a modifier and provide an explanatory note each time I report the service?*

A. Before reporting such services, you should reach an agreement with the payer about 1) its willingness to reimburse you for the service and 2) its preferred method for reporting the service.

Q. *What code should I use for reporting psychotherapy provided by telephone?*

A. There are two ways of reporting psychotherapy provided over the telephone: 1) use the code for an unlisted procedure (90899) with an explanatory note or 2) use one of the E/M codes for telephone calls (99441–99443) with an explanatory note. **The code you choose for reporting this service should be selected by agreement with the payer before you start billing for occasional or routine provision of telephone therapy. Be forewarned that many payers, including Medicare, will not reimburse for this service.**

Q. *How do I code for the time it takes me to complete commitment proceedings for a patient?*

A. You can use 90801, the code for initial psychiatric evaluations, and modifier –22, if the service requires an unusual length of time. Otherwise, you can use an E/M office service code at the appropriate level of service. If you select an office service code, only the time spent face-to-face with the patient may be used to calculate the level of service. Should the face-to-face time associated with the commitment proceedings be unusually lengthy, use the –21 modifier. Attach a brief explanatory note to the billing form.

Q. *Is there a code I can use for providing services to a patient via e-mail?*

A. Yes, there is now a CPT code for e-mail, 99444. The CPT descriptor for this code is:

> Online evaluation and management service provided by a physician to an established patient, guardian, or healthcare provider not originating from a related E/M service provided within the previous 7 days, using the Internet or similar electronic communications network.

If you want to code for e-mails with your patients, you should be sure to have some sort of written agreement with the patient and/or the insurer that this is something that will be billed for and for which you expect payment.

Codes and Documentation for Evaluation and Management Services

4

The evaluation and management (E/M) codes were introduced in the 1992 update to the fourth edition of *Physicians' Current Procedural Terminology* (CPT). These codes cover a broad range of services for patients in both inpatient and outpatient settings. In 1995 and again in 1997, the Health Care Financing Administration (now the Centers for Medicare and Medicaid Services, or CMS) published documentation guidelines to support the selection of appropriate E/M codes for services provided to Medicare beneficiaries. The major difference between the two sets of guidelines is that the 1997 set includes a single-system psychiatry examination (mental status examination) that can be fully substituted for the comprehensive, multisystem physical examination required by the 1995 guideline. Because of this, it clearly makes the most sense for mental health practitioners to use the 1997 guidelines (see Appendix E). A practical 27-page guide from CMS on how to use the documentation guidelines can be found at http://www.cms.hhs.gov/MLNProducts/downloads/eval_mgmt_serv _guide.pdf. The American Medical Association's CPT manual also provides valuable information in the introduction to its E/M section. Clinicians currently have the option of using the 1995 or 1997 CMS documentation guidelines for E/M services, although for mental health providers the 1997 version is the obvious choice.

The E/M codes are generic in the sense that they are intended to be used by all physicians, nurse-practitioners, and physician assistants and to be used in primary and specialty care alike. All of the E/M codes are available to you for reporting your services. Psychiatrists frequently ask, "Under what clinical circumstances would you use the office or other outpatient service E/M codes in lieu of the psychiatric evaluation and psychiatric therapy codes?" The decision to use one set of codes over another should be based on which code most accurately describes the services provided to the patient. The E/M codes give you flexibility for reporting your services when the service provided is more medically oriented or when counseling and coordination of care is being provided more than psychotherapy. (See p. 44 for a discussion of counseling and coordination of care).

Appendix K provides national data on the distribution of E/M codes selected by psychiatrists within the Medicare program. Please note that although there are many codes available to use for reporting services, the existence of the codes in the CPT manual does not guarantee that insurers will reimburse you for the services designated by those codes. Some insurers mandate that psychiatrists and other mental health providers only bill using the psychiatric codes (90801–90899). It is always smart to check with the payer when there are alternatives available for coding.

THE E/M CODES

- E/M codes are used by all physician specialties and all other duly licensed health providers.
- The definitions of *new patient* and *established patient* are important because of the extensive use of these terms throughout the guidelines in the E/M section. **A *new patient* is defined as one who has not received any professional services from the physician or another physician of the same specialty who belongs to the same group within the past 3 years. An *established patient* is one who has received professional services from the physician or another physician of the same specialty who belongs to the same group within the past 3 years.** When a physician is on call covering for another physician, the decision as to whether the patient is new or established is determined by the relationship of the covering physician to the physician group that has provided care to the patient for whom the coverage is now being provided. If the doctor is in the same practice, even though she has never seen the patient before, the patient is considered established. There is no distinction made between new and established patients in the emergency department.

  The other terms used in the E/M descriptors are equally as important. The terms that follow are vital to correct E/M coding (complete definitions for them can be found under Steps 4 and 5 later in this chapter):

  - Problem-focused history
  - Detailed history
  - Expanded problem-focused history
  - Comprehensive history

  - Problem-focused examination
  - Detailed examination
  - Expanded problem-focused examination
  - Comprehensive examination

- Straightforward medical decision making
- Low-complexity medical decision making
- Moderate-complexity medical decision making
- High-complexity medical decision making

- E/M codes have three to five levels of service based on increasing amounts of work.
- Most E/M codes have time elements expressed as the time "typically" spent face-to-face with the patient and/or family for outpatient care or unit floor time for inpatient care.
- For each E/M code it is noted that "Counseling and/or coordination of care with other providers or agencies is provided consistent with the nature of the problem(s) and the patient's and/or family's needs." *When this counseling and coordination of care accounts for more than 50% of the time spent, the typical time given in the code descriptor may be used for selecting the appropriate code rather than the other factors.* (See p. 44 for a discussion of counseling and co-ordination of care.)
- The 1995 and 1997 CMS documentation guidelines for E/M codes have become the basis for sometimes draconian compliance requirements for clinicians who treat Medicare beneficiaries. Commercial payers have adopted elements of the documentation system in a variable manner. *The fact is that the documentation guidelines cannot be ignored by practitioners.* To do so would place the practitioner at risk for audits, civil actions by payers, and perhaps even criminal charges and prosecution by federal agencies.

SELECTING THE LEVEL OF E/M SERVICE

The following are step-by-step instructions that guide you through the code selection process when providing services defined by E/M codes. Code selection is made based on the work performed.

Step 1: Select the Category and Subcategory of E/M Service

Table 4–1 lists the E/M services most likely to be used by psychiatrists. This table provides only a partial list of services and their codes. For the full list of E/M codes you will need to refer to the CPT manual.

TABLE 4–1. EVALUATION AND MANAGEMENT CODES MOST LIKELY TO BE USED BY
PSYCHIATRISTS

CATEGORY/SUBCATEGORY	CODE NUMBERS
Office or outpatient services	
New patient	99201–99205
Established patient	99211–99215
Hospital observational services	
Observation care discharge services	99217
Initial observation care	99218–99220
Hospital inpatient services	
Initial hospital care	99221–99223
Subsequent hospital care	99231–99233
Hospital discharge services	99238–99239
Consultations[1]	
Office consultations	99241–99245
Inpatient consultations	99251–99255
Emergency department services	
Emergency department services	99281–99288
Nursing facility services	
Initial nursing facility care	99304–99306
Subsequent nursing facility care	99307–99310
Nursing facility discharge services	99315–99316
Annual nursing facility assessment	99318
Domiciliary, rest home, or custodial care services	
New patient	99324–99328
Established patient	99334–99337
Home services	
New patient	99341–99345
Established patient	99347–99350
Team conference services	
Team conferences with patient/family[2]	99366
Team conferences without patient/family	99367
Behavior change interventions	
Smoking and tobacco use cessation	99406–99407
Alcohol and/or substance abuse structured screening and brief intervention	99408–99409
Non-face-to-face physician services[3]	
Telephone services	99441–99443
On-line medical evaluation	99444
Basic life and/or disability evaluation services	99450
Work-related or medical disability evaluation services	99455–99456

[1]Medicare no longer recognizes these codes.

[2]For team conferences with the patient/family present, physicians should use the appropriate evaluation and management code in lieu of a team conference code.

[3]Medicare covers only face-to-face services.

Step 2: Review the Descriptors and Reporting Instructions for the E/M Service Selected

Most of the categories and many of the subcategories of E/M services have special guidelines or instructions governing the use of the codes. For example, under the description of initial hospital care for a new or established patient, the CPT manual indicates that the inpatient care level of service reported by the admitting physician should include the services related to the admission that he or she provided in other sites of service as well as in the inpatient setting. E/M services that are provided on the same date in sites other than the hospital and that are related to the admission should *not* be reported separately.

Examples of Descriptors for CPT Codes Used Most Frequently by Psychiatrists
99221—Initial hospital care, per day, for the evaluation and management of a patient, which requires these three key components: • A detailed or comprehensive history • A detailed or comprehensive examination • Medical decision making that is straightforward or of low complexity Counseling and/or coordination of care with other providers or agencies is provided consistent with the nature of the problem(s) and the patient's and/or family's needs. Usually, the problem(s) requiring admission are of low severity. Physicians typically spend 30 minutes at the bedside and on the patient's hospital floor or unit.
99222—Initial hospital care, per day, for the evaluation and management of a patient, which requires these three key components: • A comprehensive history • A comprehensive examination • Medical decision making of moderate complexity Counseling and/or coordination of care with other providers or agencies is provided consistent with the nature of the problem(s) and the patient's and/or family's needs. Usually, the problem(s) requiring admission are of moderate severity. Physicians typically spend 50 minutes at the bedside and on the patient's hospital floor or unit.
99223—Initial hospital care, per day, for the evaluation and management of a patient, which requires these three key components: • A comprehensive history • A comprehensive examination • Medical decision making of high complexity Counseling and/or coordination of care with other providers or agencies is provided consistent with the nature of the problem(s) and the patient's and/or family's needs. Usually, the problem(s) requiring admission are of low severity. Physicians typically spend 70 minutes at the bedside and on the patient's hospital floor or unit.

Step 3: Review the Service Descriptors and the Requirements for the Key Components of the Selected E/M Service

Almost every category or subcategory of E/M service lists the required level of history, examination, or medical decision making for that particular code. (See the list of codes later in the chapter.)

For example, for E/M code 99223 the service descriptor is "Initial hospital care, per day, for the evaluation and management of a patient, which requires these three key components" and the code requires

- Comprehensive history
- Comprehensive examination
- Medical decision making of high complexity

Each of these components are described in Steps 4, 5, and 6.

Step 4: Determine the Extent of Work Required in Obtaining the History

The extent of the history obtained is driven by clinical judgment and the nature of the presenting problem. Four levels of work are associated with history taking. They range from the simplest to the most complete and include the components listed in the sections that follow.

The elements required for each type of history are depicted in Table 4–2. Note that each history type requires more information as you read down the left-hand column. For example, a problem-focused history requires the documentation of the chief complaint (CC) and a brief history of present illness (HPI), and a detailed history requires the documentation of a CC, an extended HPI, an extended review of systems (ROS), and a pertinent past, family, and/or social history (PFSH).

The extent of information gathered for a history is dependent on clinical judgment and the nature of the presenting problem. Documentation of patient history includes some or all of the following elements.

A. CHIEF COMPLAINT (CC)

The chief complaint is a concise statement that describes the symptom, problem, condition, diagnosis, or reason for the patient encounter. It is usually stated in the patient's own words. For example, "I am anxious, feel depressed, and am tired all the time."

B. HISTORY OF PRESENT ILLNESS (HPI)

The history of present illness is a chronological description of the development of the patient's present illness from the first sign and/or symptom or from the previous encounter to the present. HPI elements are:

- Location (e.g., feeling depressed)
- Quality (e.g., hopeless, helpless, worried)
- Severity (e.g., 8 on a scale of 1 to 10)
- Duration (e.g., it started 2 weeks ago)

TABLE 4–2. ELEMENTS REQUIRED FOR EACH TYPE OF HISTORY

TYPE OF HISTORY	CHIEF COMPLAINT	HISTORY OF PRESENT ILLNESS	REVIEW OF SYSTEMS	PAST, FAMILY, AND/OR SOCIAL HISTORY
Problem focused	Required	Brief	N/A	N/A
Expanded problem focused	Required	Brief	Problem pertinent	N/A
Detailed	Required	Extended	Extended	Pertinent
Comprehensive	Required	Extended	Complete	Complete

- Timing (e.g., worse in the morning)
- Context (e.g., fired from job)
- Modifying factors (e.g., feels better with people around)
- Associated signs and symptoms (e.g., loss of appetite, loss of weight, loss of sexual interest)

There are two types of HPIs, *brief* and *extended:*

1. *Brief* includes documentation of one to three HPI elements. In the following example, three HPI elements—location, severity, and duration—are documented:

   - CC: Patient complains of depression.
   - Brief HPI: Patient complains of feeling severely depressed for the past 2 weeks.

2. *Extended* includes documentation of at least four HPI elements or the status of at least three chronic or inactive conditions. In the following example, five HPI elements—location, severity, duration, context, and modifying factors—are documented:

   - CC: Patient complains of depression.
   - Extended HPI: Patient complains of feelings of depression for the past 2 weeks. Lost his job 3 weeks ago. Is worried about finances. Trouble sleeping, loss of appetite, and loss of sexual interest. Rates depressive feelings as 8/10.

C. REVIEW OF SYSTEMS (ROS)

The review of systems is an inventory of body systems obtained by asking a series of questions in order to identify signs and/or symptoms that the patient may be experiencing or has experienced. The following systems are recognized:

- Constitutional (e.g., temperature, weight, height, blood pressure)
- Eyes
- Ears, nose, mouth, throat
- Cardiovascular
- Respiratory

- Gastrointestinal
- Genitourinary
- Musculoskeletal
- Integumentary (skin and/or breast)
- Neurological
- Psychiatric
- Endocrine
- Hematologic/Lymphatic
- Allergic/Immunologic

There are three levels of ROS:

1. *Problem pertinent,* which inquires about the system directly related to the problem identified in the HPI. In the following example, one system—psychiatric—is reviewed:

   - CC: Depression.
   - ROS: Positive for appetite loss and weight loss of 5 pounds (gastrointestinal/constitutional).

2. *Extended,* which inquires about the system directly related to the problem(s) identified in the HPI and a limited number (two to nine) of additional systems. In the following example, two systems—constitutional and neurological—are reviewed:

   - CC: Depression.
   - ROS: Patient reports a 5-lb weight loss over 3 weeks and problems sleeping, with early morning wakefulness.

3. *Complete,* which inquires about the system(s) directly related to the problem(s) identified in the HPI plus all additional (minimum of 10) body systems. In the following example, 10 signs and symptoms are reviewed:

   - CC: Patient complains of depression.
   - ROS:
     a. Constitutional: Weight loss of 5 lb over 3 weeks
     b. Eyes: No complaints
     c. Ear, nose, mouth, throat: No complaints
     d. Cardiovascular: No complaints
     e. Respiratory: No complaints
     f. Gastrointestinal: Appetite loss
     g. Urinary: No complaints
     h. Skin: No complaints
     i. Neurological: Trouble falling asleep, early morning awakening
     j. Psychiatric: Depression and loss of sexual interest

D. PAST, FAMILY, AND/OR SOCIAL HISTORY (PFSH)

There are three basic history areas required for a complete PFSH:

1. Past medical/psychiatric history: Illnesses, operations, injuries, treatments

2. Family history: Family medical history, events, hereditary illnesses
3. Social history: Age-appropriate review of past and current activities

The data elements of a textbook psychiatric history, listed below, are substantially more complete than the elements required to meet the threshold for a comprehensive or complete PFSH:

- Family history
- Birth and upbringing
- Milestones
- Past medical history
- Past psychiatric history
- Educational history
- Vocational history
- Religious background
- Dating and marital history
- Military history
- Legal history

The two levels of PFSH are:

1. *Pertinent,* which is a review of the history areas directly related to the problem(s) identified in the HPI. The pertinent PFSH must document one item from any of the three history areas. In the following example, the patient's past psychiatric history is reviewed as it relates to the current HPI:

- Patient has a history of a depressive episode 10 years ago successfully treated with Prozac. Episode lasted 3 months.

2. *Complete.* At least one specific item from two of the three basic history areas must be documented for a complete PFSH for the following categories of E/M services:

- Office or other outpatient services, established patient
- Emergency department
- Domiciliary care, established patient
- Home care, established patient

At least one specific item from each of the three basic history areas must be documented for the following categories of E/M services:

- Office or other outpatient services, new patient
- Hospital observation services
- Hospital inpatient services, initial care
- Consultations
- Comprehensive nursing facility assessments
- Domiciliary care, new patient
- Home care, new patient

Documentation of History.   Once the level of history is determined, documentation of that level of HPI, ROS, and PFSH is accomplished by listing the required number of elements for each of the three components (see Table 4–3).

TABLE 4–3. PATIENT HISTORY TAKING

ELEMENT — Level of history is achieved when all four of the four criteria for each element are completed for that level.	LEVELS			
	Problem focused	Expanded problem focused	Detailed	Comprehensive
CRITERIA				
Chief complaint (always required): Should include a brief statement, usually in the patient's own words; symptom(s); problem; condition; diagnosis; and reason for the encounter	Chief complaint	Chief complaint	Chief complaint	Chief complaint
History of the present illness: A chronological description of the development of the patient's present illness • Associated signs and symptoms • Context • Duration • Location • Modifying factors • Quality • Severity • Timing	Brief, one to three bullets	Brief, one to three bullets	Extended, four or more bullets	Extended, four or more bullets
Review of systems: An inventory of body systems to identify signs and/or symptoms • Allergic, immunologic • Cardiovascular • Constitutional (fever, weight loss) • Ears, nose, mouth, throat • Endocrine • Eyes • Gastrointestinal • Genitourinary • Hematologic, lymphatic • Integumentary (skin, breast) • Musculoskeletal • Neurological • Psychiatric • Respiratory	None	Pertinent to problem, one system	Extended, two to nine systems	Complete, 10 or more systems or some systems with statement "all others negative"
Past, family, and/or social history: Chronological review of relevant data • Past history: Illnesses, operations, injuries, treatments • Family history: Family medical history, events, hereditary illnesses • Social history: Age-appropriate review of past and current activities	None	None	Pertinent, one history area	Complete, two or three history areas

An ROS and/or PFSH taken during an earlier visit need not be rerecorded if there is evidence that it has been reviewed and any changes to the previous information have been noted. The ROS may be obtained by ancillary staff or may be provided on forms completed by the patient. The clinician must review the ROS, supplement and/or confirm the pertinent positives and negatives, and document the review. By doing so, the clinician takes medical-legal responsibility for the accuracy of the data. If the condition of the patient prevents the clinician from obtaining a history, the clinician should describe the patient's condition or the circumstances that precluded obtaining the history. **Failure to provide and record the required number of elements of the ROS for the level of history designated is the most frequently cited deficiency in audits of clinicians' mental health records.**

See Appendix H for examples of templates that provide a structure that will ensure that the clinician's note and documentation requirements are met. The Attending Physician Admitting Note template for initial hospital case with a complete history qualifies for a comprehensive level of history. The Attending Physician Subsequent Care template for inpatient subsequent care or outpatient established care contains the required elements for three levels of inpatient subsequent care or five levels of outpatient established care.

Step 5: Determine the Extent of Work in Performing the Examination

The mental status examination of a patient is considered a single system examination. The elements of the examination are provided in Table 4–4. This definition of what composes a mental status examination was jointly published by the American Medical Association and Health Care Financing Administration (now CMS) in 1997. There are four levels of work associated with performing a mental status examination.

Table 4–4 is a summary of the four levels of examination and the number of bullets (elements) required for each level. Template examples for the mental status examination are illustrated in Appendix H. **Failure to provide and record the required number of constitutional elements (including vital signs) is the second most frequently cited deficiency in audits of clinicians' medical records.**

Step 6: Determine the Complexity of Medical Decision Making

Medical decision making is the complex task of establishing a diagnosis and selecting treatment and management options. **Medical decision making is closely tied to the nature of the presenting problem.** A *presenting problem* is a disease, symptom, sign, finding, complaint, or other reason for the encounter having been initiated.

- *Minimal*—A problem that may or may not require physician presence, but the services provided are under physician supervision.
- *Self-limited or minor*—A problem that is transient, runs a definite course, and is unlikely to permanently alter health status.

TABLE 4–4. CONTENT AND DOCUMENTATION REQUIREMENTS FOR THE SINGLE SYSTEM PSYCHIATRIC EXAMINATION

SYSTEM/BODY AREA AND ELEMENTS OF EXAMINATION	CRITERIA			
	One to five elements identified by a bullet	At least six elements identified by a bullet	At least nine elements identified by a bullet	All elements identified by a bullet
Constitutional • Measurement of *any three of the following seven vital signs* (may be measured and recorded by ancillary staff): 1. Sitting or standing blood pressure 2. Supine blood pressure 3. Pulse rate and regularity 4. Respiration 5. Temperature 6. Height 7. Weight • General appearance of patient (e.g., development, nutrition, body habitus, deformities, attention to grooming) **Musculoskeletal** • Assessment of muscle strength and tone • Examination of gait and station **Psychiatric** *Description of patient's* • Speech, including rate, volume, articulation, coherence, and spontaneity, with notation of abnormalities (e.g., perseveration, paucity of language) • Thought processes, including rate of thoughts, content of thoughts (e.g., logical versus illogical, tangential), abstract reasoning, and computation • Associations (e.g., loose tangential, circumstantial, intact) • Abnormal psychotic thoughts, including hallucinations, delusions, preoccupation with violence, homicidal or suicidal ideation, and obsessions • Mood and affect (e.g., depression, anxiety, agitation, hypomania, lability) • Judgment (e.g., concerning everyday activities and social situations) and insight (e.g., concerning psychiatric condition) *Complete mental status examination, including* • Orientation to time, place, and person • Recent and remote memory • Attention span and concentration • Language (e.g., naming objects, repeating phrases) • Fund of knowledge (e.g., awareness of current events, past history, vocabulary)				
Level of examination is achieved when the number of criteria specified for a given level is met	Problem focused	Expanded problem focused	Detailed	Comprehensive

Source. Centers for Medicare and Medicaid Services 1997 Guidelines for Documentation of Evaluation and Management Services.

- *Low severity*—A problem of low morbidity, no risk of mortality, and expectation of full recovery with no residual functional incapacity.
- *Moderate severity*—A problem with moderate risk of morbidity and/or mortality without treatment, uncertain outcome, and probability of prolonged functional impairment.
- *High severity*—A problem of high to extreme morbidity without treatment, moderate to high risk of mortality without treatment, and/or probability of severe, prolonged functional impairment.

Medical decision making is based on three sets of data:

1. *The number of diagnoses and management options:* As specified in Table 4–5, this is the first step in determining the type of medical decision making.

TABLE 4–5. NUMBER OF DIAGNOSES AND MANAGEMENT OPTIONS

	MINIMAL	LIMITED	MULTIPLE	EXTENSIVE
Diagnoses	One established	One established [and] one rule-out or differential	Two rule-out or differential	More than two rule-out or differential
Problem(s)	Improved	Stable Resolving	Unstable Failing to change	Worsening Marked change
Management options	One or two	Two or three	Three changes in treatment plan	Four or more changes in treatment plan

Note. To qualify for a given type of decision making, two of three elements must be met or exceeded.

2. *The amount and/or complexity of medical records, diagnostic tests, and/or other information that must be obtained, reviewed, and analyzed:* Table 4–6 lists the elements and criteria that determine the level of decision making for this set of data.

TABLE 4–6. AMOUNT AND/OR COMPLEXITY OF DATA TO BE REVIEWED

	MINIMAL	LIMITED	MODERATE	EXTENSIVE
Medical data	One source	Two sources	Three sources	Multiple sources
Diagnostic tests	Two	Three	Four	More than four
Review of results	Confirmatory review	Confirmation of results with another physician	Results discussed with physician performing tests	Unexpected results, contradictory reviews, requires additional reviews

Note. To qualify for a given type of decision making, two of three elements must be met or exceeded.

3. *Risk of complications and/or morbidity or mortality as well as comorbidities:* As with the two previous tables, Table 4–7 provides the elements and criteria used to rate this particular data set.

TABLE 4–7. TABLE OF RISK

LEVEL OF RISK	PRESENTING PROBLEM(S)	DIAGNOSTIC PROCEDURE(S) ORDERED	MANAGEMENT OPTIONS SELECTED
Minimal	One self-limited problem (e.g., medication side effect)	Laboratory tests requiring venipuncture Urinalysis	Reassurance
Low	Two or more self-limited or minor problems or one stable, chronic illness (e.g., well-controlled depression) or acute uncomplicated illness (e.g., exacerbation of anxiety disorder)	Psychological testing Skull film	Psychotherapy Environmental intervention (e.g., agency, school, vocational placement) Referral for consultation (e.g., physician, social worker)
Moderate	One or more chronic illness with mild exacerbation, progression, or side effects of treatment or two or more stable chronic illnesses or undiagnosed new problem with uncertain prognosis (e.g., psychosis)	Electroencephalogram Neuropsychological testing	Prescription drug management Open-door seclusion Electroconvulsive therapy, inpatient, outpatient, routine; no comorbid medical conditions
High	One or more chronic illnesses with severe exacerbation, progression, or side effect of treatment (e.g., schizophrenia) or acute illness with threat to life (e.g., suicidal or homicidal ideation)	Lumbar puncture Suicide risk assessment	Drug therapy requiring intensive monitoring (e.g., tapering diazepam for patient in withdrawal) Closed-door seclusion Suicide observation Electroconvulsive therapy; patient has comorbid medical condition (e.g., cardiovascular disease) Rapid intramuscular neuroleptic administration Pharmacological restraint

Source.   Modified from CMS 1997 Guidelines for Psychiatry Single System Exam.

DETERMINING THE OVERALL LEVEL OF MEDICAL DECISION MAKING

Table 4–8 provides a grid that includes the components of the three preceding tables and level of complexity for each of those three components. The overall level of decision making is decided by placing the level of each of the three components into the appropriate box in a manner that allows them to be summed up to rate the overall decision making as *straightforward, low complexity, moderate complexity,* or *high complexity.*

DOCUMENTATION

The use of templates, either preprinted forms or embedded in an electronic patient record (see Appendix H), is an efficient means of addressing the documentation of decision making. Rather than counting or scoring the elements of the three components and actually filling out a grid like the one in the Table 4–8, a template can be constructed in collaboration with the compliance officer of your practice or institution to include prompts that capture the required data necessary to document complexity. Solo practitioners may require the assistance of their specialty association or a consultant to develop appropriate templates.

The templates in Appendix H fulfill the documentation requirements for both clinical and compliance needs. The fifth page of the Attending Physician Admission Note template includes all of the elements necessary for addressing Step 6 of the E/M decision-making process. Similarly, the second page of the daily note for inpatient or outpatient care also includes the elements for documenting medical decision making.

Remember: Clinically, there is a close relationship between the nature of the presenting problem and the complexity of medical decision making. For example:

- Patient A comes in for a prescription refill—straightforward decision making
- Patient B presents with suicidal ideation—decision making of high complexity

TABLE 4–8. ELEMENTS AND TYPE OF MEDICAL DECISION MAKING

	TYPE OF DECISION MAKING			
	Straightforward	Low complexity	Moderate complexity	High complexity
Number of diagnoses or management options (Table 4–5)	Minimal	Limited	Multiple	Extensive
Amount and/or complexity of data to be reviewed (Table 4–6)	Minimal or none	Limited	Moderate	Extensive
Risk of complications and/or morbidity or mortality (Table 4–7)	Minimal	Low	Moderate	High

Note. To qualify for a given type of decision making, two of three elements must be met or exceeded.

Step 7: Select the Appropriate Level of E/M Service

As noted earlier, each category of E/M service has three to five levels of work associated with it. Each level of work has a descriptor of the service and the required extent of the three key components of work. For example:

99223   **Descriptor:** Initial hospital care, per day for the evaluation and management of a patient, which requires these three key components:

- A comprehensive history
- A comprehensive examination
- Medical decision making that is of high complexity

For new patients, the three key components (history, examination, and medical decision making) must meet or exceed the stated requirements to qualify for each level of service for office visits, initial hospital care, office consultations, initial inpatient consultations, confirmatory consultations, emergency department services, comprehensive nursing facility assessments, domiciliary care, and home services.

For established patients, two of the three key components (history, examination, and medical decision making) must meet or exceed the stated requirements to qualify for each level of service for office visits, subsequent hospital care, follow-up inpatient consultations, subsequent nursing facility care, domiciliary care, and home care.

WHEN COUNSELING AND COORDINATION OF CARE ACCOUNT FOR MORE THAN 50% OF THE FACE-TO-FACE PHYSICIAN–PATIENT ENCOUNTER

When counseling and coordination of care account for more than 50% of the face-to-face physician–patient encounter, then time becomes the key or controlling factor in selecting the level of service. Note that counseling or coordination of care must be documented in the medical record. The definitions of counseling, coordination of care, and time follow.

Counseling is a discussion with a patient or the patient's family concerning one or more of the following issues:

- Diagnostic results, impressions, and/or recommended diagnostic studies
- Prognosis
- Risks and benefits of management (treatment) options
- Instructions for management (treatment) and/or follow-up
- Importance of adherence to chosen management (treatment) options
- Risk factor reduction
- Patient and family education

Coordination of care is not specifically defined in the E/M section of the CPT manual. A working definition of the term could be as follows: Services provided by the physician responsible for the direct care of a patient when he or she coordinates or controls access to care or initiates or supervises other healthcare services needed by the patient. Outpatient coordination of care must be provided face-to-face with the patient. Coordination of care with other providers or agencies without the patient being present on that day is reported with the case management codes.

TIME

For the purpose of selecting the level of service, time has two definitions.

1. For office and other outpatient visits and office consultations, *intraservice time* (time spent by the clinician providing services with the patient and/or family present) is defined as face-to-face time. Pre- and post-encounter time (non-face-to-face time) is not included in the average times listed under each level of service for either office or outpatient consultative services. The work associated with pre- and post-encounter time has been calculated into the total work effort provided by the physician for that service.

2. Time spent providing inpatient and nursing facility services is defined as *unit/floor time*. Unit/floor time includes all work provided to the patient while the psychiatrist is on the unit. This includes the following:

   - Direct patient contact (face-to-face)
   - Review of charts
   - Writing of orders
   - Writing of progress notes
   - Reviewing test results
   - Meeting with the treatment team
   - Telephone calls
   - Meeting with the family or other caregivers
   - Patient and family education

Work completed before and after direct patient contact and presence on the unit/floor, such as reviewing X-rays in another part of the hospital, has been included in the calculation of the total work provided by the physician for that service. Unit/floor time may be used to select the level of inpatient services by matching the total unit/floor time to the average times listed for each level of inpatient service. For instance:

99221   **Descriptor:** Initial hospital care, per day, for the evaluation and management of a patient, which requires these three key components:

- A detailed or comprehensive history
- A detailed or comprehensive examination
- Medical decision making that is straightforward or of low complexity

Counseling and/or coordination of care with other providers or agencies are provided consistent with the nature of the problem(s) and the patient's and/or family's needs.

Usually, the problem(s) requiring admission are of low severity. Physicians typically spend 30 minutes at the bedside and on the patient's hospital floor or unit.

Table 4–9 provides an example of an auditor's worksheet employed in making the decision of whether to use time in selecting the level of service. The three questions are prompts that assist the auditor (usually a nurse reviewer) in assessing whether the clinician 1) documented the length of time of the patient encounter, 2) described the counseling or coordination of care, and 3) indicated that more than half of the encounter time was for counseling or coordination of care.

> **Important:** If you elect to report the level of service based on counseling and/or coordination of care, the total length of time of the encounter should be documented and the record should describe the counseling and/or services or activities performed to coordinate care.

TABLE 4–9. Choosing Level Based on Time

	YES	NO
Does documentation reveal total time? Time: Face-to-face in outpatient setting; unit/floor in inpatient setting		
Does documentation describe the content of counseling or coordinating care?		
Does documentation suggest that more than half of the total time was counseling or coordinating of care?		

Note.   If all answers are yes, select level based on time.

For examples and vignettes of code selection in specific clinical settings, see Chapter 5.

EVALUATION AND MANAGEMENT CODES MOST LIKELY TO BE USED BY PSYCHIATRISTS AND OTHER APPROPRIATELY LICENSED MENTAL HEALTH PROFESSIONALS

It is vital to read the explanatory notes in the CPT manual for an accurate understanding of when each of these codes should be used.

> **Note:** For each of the following codes it is noted that: "Counseling and/or coordination of care with other providers or agencies is provided consistent with the nature of the problem(s) and the patient's and/or family's needs." As stated earlier, when this counseling and coordination of care accounts for more than 50% of the time spent, the typical time given in the code descriptor may be used for selecting the appropriate code rather than the other factors.

Office or Other Outpatient Services

NEW PATIENT

99201—The three following components are required:

- Problem-focused history
- Problem-focused examination
- Medical decision making that is straightforward

Presenting problem(s): Self-limited or minor
Typical time: 10 minutes face-to-face with patient and/or family

99202—The three following components are required:

- Expanded problem-focused history
- Expanded problem-focused examination
- Medical decision making that is straightforward

Presenting problem(s): Low to moderate severity
Typical time: 20 minutes face-to-face with patient and/or family

99203—The three following components are required:

- Detailed history
- Detailed examination
- Medical decision making of low complexity

Presenting problem(s): Moderate severity
Typical time: 30 minutes face-to-face with patient and/or family

99204—The three following components are required:

- Comprehensive history
- Comprehensive examination
- Medical decision making of moderate complexity

Presenting problem(s): Moderate to high severity
Typical time: 45 minutes face-to-face with patient and/or family

99205—The three following components are required:

- Comprehensive history
- Comprehensive examination
- Medical decision making of high complexity

Presenting problem(s): Moderate to high severity
Typical time: 60 minutes face-to-face with patient and/or family

ESTABLISHED PATIENT

99211—This code is used for a service that may not require the presence of a physician. Presenting problems are minimal, and 5 minutes is the typical time that would be spent performing or supervising these services.

***99212*—Two of the three following components are required:**

- Problem-focused history
- Problem-focused examination
- Medical decision making that is straightforward

  Presenting problem(s): Self-limited or minor
  Typical time: 10 minutes face-to-face with patient and/or family

 ***99213*—Two of the three following components are required:**

- Expanded problem-focused history
- Expanded problem-focused examination
- Medical decision making of low complexity

  Presenting problem(s): Low to moderate severity
  Typical time: 15 minutes face-to-face with patient and/or family

***99214*—Two of the three following components are required:**

- Detailed history
- Detailed examination
- Medical decision making of moderate complexity

  Presenting problem(s): Moderate to high severity
  Typical time: 25 minutes face-to-face with patient and/or family

***99215*—Two of the three following components are required:**

- Comprehensive history
- Comprehensive examination
- Medical decision making of high complexity

  Presenting problem(s): Moderate to high severity
  Typical time: 40 minutes face-to-face with patient and/or family

Hospital Observational Services

OBSERVATION CARE DISCHARGE SERVICES

***99217*—This code is used to report all services provided on discharge from "observation status" if the discharge occurs after the initial date of "observation status."**

INITIAL OBSERVATION CARE

***99218*—The three following components are required:**

- Detailed or comprehensive history
- Detailed or comprehensive examination
- Medical decision making of straightforward or of low complexity

  Presenting problem(s): Low severity
  Typical time: None listed

99219—**The three following components are required:**

- Comprehensive history
- Comprehensive examination
- Medical decision making of moderate complexity

Presenting problem(s): Moderate severity
Typical time: None listed

99220—**The three following components are required:**

- Comprehensive history
- Comprehensive examination
- Medical decision making of high complexity

Presenting problem(s): High severity
Typical time: None listed

Hospital Inpatient Services

Services provided in a partial hospitalization setting would also use these codes. (With the elimination of the consultation codes as of January 1, 2010, CMS has created a new modifier A1, that is used to denote the admitting physician.)

INITIAL HOSPITAL CARE FOR NEW OR ESTABLISHED PATIENT

99221—**The three following components are required:**

- Detailed or comprehensive history
- Detailed or comprehensive examination
- Medical decision making that is straightforward or of low complexity

Presenting problem(s): Low severity
Typical time: 30 minutes at the bedside or on the patient's floor or unit

99222—**The three following components are required:**

- Comprehensive history
- Comprehensive examination
- Medical decision making of moderate complexity

Presenting problem(s): Moderate severity
Typical time: 50 minutes at the bedside or on the patient's floor or unit

99223—**The three following components are required:**

- Comprehensive history
- Comprehensive examination
- Medical decision making of high complexity

Presenting problem(s): High severity
Typical time: 70 minutes at the bedside or on the patient's floor or unit

SUBSEQUENT HOSPITAL CARE

99231—Two of the three following components are required:

- Problem-focused interval history
- Problem-focused examination
- Medical decision making that is straightforward or of low complexity

   Presenting problem(s): Patient usually stable, recovering, or improving
   Typical time: 15 minutes at the bedside or on the patient's floor or unit

99232—Two of the three following components are required:

- Expanded problem-focused interval history
- Expanded problem-focused examination
- Medical decision making of moderate complexity

   Presenting problem(s): Patient responding inadequately to therapy or has developed a minor complication
   Typical time: 25 minutes at the bedside or on the patient's floor or unit

99233—Two of the three following components are required:

- Detailed interval history
- Detailed examination
- Medical decision making of high complexity

   Presenting problem(s): Patient unstable or has developed a significant new problem
   Typical time: 35 minutes at the bedside or on the patient's floor or unit

HOSPITAL DISCHARGE SERVICES

99238—Time: 30 minutes or less

99239—Time: More than 30 minutes

Consultations

Medicare no longer pays for the consultation codes. When coding for Medicare or for commercial carriers that have followed Medicare's lead, 90801 may be used for both inpatient and outpatient consults. Psychiatrists who choose to use E/M codes to report outpatient consults should use the outpatient new patient codes (99201–99205). For inpatient consults, the codes to use are hospital inpatient services, initial hospital care for new or established patients (99221–99223). For consults in nursing homes, initial nursing facility care codes should be used (99304–99306); if the consult is of low complexity, the subsequent nursing facility codes may be used (99307–99310). As with all E/M codes, the selection of the specific code is based on the complexity of the case and the amount of work required. Medicare has created a new modifier, A1, to denote the admitting physician so that more than one physician may use the initial hospital care codes.

OFFICE OR OTHER OUTPATIENT CONSULTATIONS

99241—The three following components are required:

- Problem-focused history
- Problem-focused examination
- Medical decision making that is straightforward

Presenting problem(s): Self-limited or minor
Typical time: 15 minutes face-to-face with patient and/or family

99242—The three following components are required:

- Expanded problem-focused history
- Expanded problem-focused examination
- Medical decision making that is straightforward

Presenting problem(s): Low severity
Typical time: 30 minutes face-to-face with patient and/or family

99243—The three following components are required:

- Detailed history
- Detailed examination
- Medical decision making of low complexity

Presenting problem(s): Moderate severity
Typical time: 40 minutes face-to-face with patient and/or family

99244—The three following components are required:

- Comprehensive history
- Comprehensive examination
- Medical decision making of moderate complexity

Presenting problem(s): Moderate to high severity
Typical time: 60 minutes face-to-face with patient and/or family

99245—The three following components are required:

- Comprehensive history
- Comprehensive examination
- Medical decision making of high complexity

Presenting problem(s): Moderate to high severity
Typical time: 80 minutes face-to-face with patient and/or family

INPATIENT CONSULTATIONS

99251—The three following components are required:

- Problem-focused history
- Problem-focused examination
- Medical decision making that is straightforward

Presenting problem(s): Self-limited or minor
Typical time: 20 minutes at the bedside or on the patient's floor or unit

99252—The three following components are required:

- Expanded problem-focused history
- Expanded problem-focused examination
- Medical decision making that is straightforward

   Presenting problem(s): Low severity
   Typical time: 40 minutes at the bedside or on the patient's floor or unit

99253—The three following components are required:

- Detailed history
- Detailed examination
- Medical decision making of low complexity

   Presenting problem(s): Moderate severity
   Typical time: 55 minutes at the bedside or on the patient's floor or unit

99254—The three following components are required:

- Comprehensive history
- Comprehensive examination
- Medical decision making of moderate complexity

   Presenting problem(s): Moderate to high severity
   Typical time: 80 minutes at the bedside or on the patient's floor or unit

99255—The three following components are required:

- Comprehensive history
- Comprehensive examination
- Medical decision making of moderate complexity

   Presenting problem(s): Moderate to high severity
   Typical time: 110 minutes at the bedside or on the patient's floor or unit

Emergency Department Services

No distinction is made between new and established patients in this setting. There are no typical times provided for emergency E/M services.

99281—The three following components are required:

- Problem-focused history
- Problem-focused examination
- Medical decision making that is straightforward

   Presenting problem(s): Self-limited or minor

99282—The three following components are required:

- Expanded problem-focused history
- Expanded problem-focused examination
- Medical decision making of low complexity

   Presenting problem(s): Low or moderate severity

99283—The three following components are required:

- Expanded problem-focused history
- Expanded problem-focused examination
- Medical decision making of moderate complexity

Presenting problem(s): Moderate severity

99284—The three following components are required:

- Detailed history
- Detailed examination
- Medical decision making of moderate complexity

Presenting problem(s): High severity

99285—The three following components are required:

- Comprehensive history
- Comprehensive examination
- Medical decision making of high complexity

Presenting problem(s): High severity and pose(s) an immediate and significant threat to life or physiological function

Nursing Facility Services

INITIAL NURSING FACILITY CARE

99304—The three following components are required:

- Detailed or comprehensive history
- Detailed or comprehensive examination
- Medical decision making that is straightforward or of low complexity

Problem(s) requiring admission: Low severity
Typical time: 25 minutes with patient and/or family or caregiver

99305—The three following components are required:

- Comprehensive history
- Comprehensive examination
- Medical decision making of moderate complexity

Problem(s) requiring admission: Moderate severity
Typical time: 35 minutes with patient and/or family or caregiver

99306—The three following components are required:

- Comprehensive history
- Comprehensive examination
- Medical decision making of high complexity

Problem(s) requiring admission: High severity
Typical time: 45 minutes with patient and/or family or caregiver

SUBSEQUENT NURSING FACILITY CARE

99307—Two of the three following components are required:

- Problem-focused interval history
- Problem-focused examination
- Medical decision making that is straightforward

   Presenting problem(s): Patient usually stable, recovering, or improving
   Typical time: 10 minutes with patient and/or family or caregiver

99308—Two of the three following components are required:

- Expanded problem-focused interval history
- Expanded problem-focused examination
- Medical decision making of low complexity

   Presenting problem(s): Patient usually responding inadequately to therapy or has developed a minor complication
   Typical time: 15 minutes with patient and/or family or caregiver

99309—Two of the three following components are required:

- Detailed interval history
- Detailed examination
- Medical decision making of moderate complexity

   Presenting problem(s): Patient usually has developed a significant complication or a significant new problem
   Typical time: 25 minutes with patient and/or family or caregiver

99310—Two of the three following components are required:

- Comprehensive interval history
- Comprehensive examination
- Medical decision making of high complexity

   Presenting problem(s): Patient may be unstable or may have developed a significant new problem requiring immediate physician attention
   Typical time: 35 minutes with patient and/or family or caregiver

NURSING FACILITY DISCHARGE SERVICES

99315—Time: 30 minutes or less

99316—Time: More than 30 minutes

ANNUAL NURSING FACILITY ASSESSMENT

99318—The three following components are required:

- Detailed interval history
- Comprehensive examination
- Medical decision making of low to moderate complexity

   Presenting problem(s): Patient usually stable, recovering, or improving
   Typical time: 30 minutes with patient and/or family or caregiver

Domiciliary, Rest Home, or Custodial Care Services

The following codes are used to report E/M services in a facility that provides room, board, and other personal services, usually on a long-term basis. They are also used in assisted living facilities.

NEW PATIENT

99324—The three following components are required:

- Problem-focused history
- Problem-focused examination
- Medical decision making that is straightforward

Presenting problem(s): Low severity
Typical time: 20 minutes with patient and/or family or caregiver

99325—The three following components are required:

- Expanded problem-focused history
- Expanded problem-focused examination
- Medical decision making of low complexity

Presenting problem(s): Moderate severity
Typical time: 30 minutes with patient and/or family or caregiver

99326—The three following components are required:

- Detailed history
- Detailed examination
- Medical decision making of moderate complexity

Presenting problem(s): Moderate to high severity
Typical time: 45 minutes with patient and/or family or caregiver

99327—The three following components are required:

- Comprehensive history
- Comprehensive examination
- Medical decision making of moderate complexity

Presenting problem(s): High severity
Typical time: 60 minutes with patient and/or family or caregiver

99328—The three following components are required:

- Comprehensive history
- Comprehensive examination
- Medical decision making of high complexity

Presenting problem(s): Patient usually has developed a significant new problem requiring immediate physician attention
Typical time: 75 minutes with patient and/or family or caregiver

ESTABLISHED PATIENT

99334—Two of the three following components are required:

- Problem-focused interval history
- Problem-focused examination
- Medical decision making that is straightforward

  Presenting problem(s): Self-limited or minor
  Typical time: 15 minutes with patient and/or family or caregiver

99335—Two of the three following components are required:

- Expanded problem-focused interval history
- Expanded problem-focused examination
- Medical decision making of low complexity

  Presenting problem(s): Low to moderate severity
  Typical time: 25 minutes with patient and/or family or caregiver

99336—Two of the three following components are required:

- Detailed interval history
- Detailed examination
- Medical decision making of moderate complexity

  Presenting problem(s): Moderate to high severity
  Typical time: 40 minutes with patient and/or family or caregiver

99337—Two of the three following components are required:

- Comprehensive interval history
- Comprehensive examination
- Medical decision making of moderate to high complexity

  Presenting problem(s): Patient may be unstable or has developed a significant new problem requiring immediate physician attention
  Typical time: 60 minutes with patient and/or family or caregiver

Home Services

These codes are used for E/M services provided to a patient in a private residence, in other words, for home visits.

NEW PATIENT

99341—The three following components are required:

- Problem-focused history
- Problem-focused examination
- Medical decision making that is straightforward

  Presenting problem(s): Low severity
  Typical time: 20 minutes face-to-face with patient and/or family

99342—The three following components are required:

- Expanded problem-focused history
- Expanded problem-focused examination
- Medical decision making of low complexity

Presenting problem(s): Moderate severity
Typical time: 30 minutes face-to-face with patient and/or family

99343—The three following components are required:

- Detailed history
- Detailed examination
- Medical decision making of moderate complexity

Presenting problem(s): Moderate to high severity
Typical time: 45 minutes face-to-face with patient and/or family

99344—The three following components are required:

- Comprehensive history
- Comprehensive examination
- Medical decision making of moderate complexity

Presenting problem(s): High severity
Typical time: 60 minutes face-to-face with patient and/or family

99345—The three following components are required:

- Comprehensive history
- Comprehensive examination
- Medical decision making of high complexity

Presenting problem(s): Patient unstable or has developed a significant new problem that requires immediate physician attention
Typical time: 75 minutes face-to-face with patient and/or family

ESTABLISHED PATIENT

99347—Two of the three following components are required:

- Problem-focused interval history
- Problem-focused examination
- Medical decision making that is straightforward

Presenting problem(s): Self-limited or minor
Typical time: 15 minutes face-to-face with patient and/or family

99348—Two of the three following components are required:

- Expanded problem-focused interval history
- Expanded problem-focused examination
- Medical decision making of low complexity

Presenting problem(s): Low to moderate severity
Typical time: 25 minutes face-to-face with patient and/or family

99349—Two of the three following components are required:

- Detailed interval history
- Detailed examination
- Medical decision making of moderate complexity

    Presenting problem(s): Moderate to high severity
    Typical time: 40 minutes face-to-face with patient and/or family

99350—Two of the three following components are required:

- Comprehensive interval history
- Comprehensive examination
- Medical decision making of moderate to high complexity

    Presenting problem(s): Moderate to high severity—patient may be unstable or may have developed a significant new problem requiring immediate physician attention
    Typical time: 60 minutes face-to-face with patient and/or family

Case Management Services

MEDICAL TEAM CONFERENCES

99366—To be used when patient and/or family is present*
Physicians should use the appropriate code from the "Evaluation and Management" section when reporting this service.

99367—To be used when there is no face-to-face contact with the patient and/or family

Preventive Medicine Services

COUNSELING RISK FACTOR REDUCTION AND BEHAVIOR CHANGE INTERVENTION

99406—Time: 3–10 minutes

99407—Time: More than 10 minutes

99408—Time: 15–30 minutes, includes the administration of an alcohol and/or substance abuse screening tool and brief intervention

99409—Time: 30 minutes or more

NON-FACE-TO-FACE SERVICES

Medicare does not pay for these.

Telephone Services

99441—Time: 5–10 minutes of medical discussion

99442—Time: 11–20 minutes of medical discussion

99443—Time: 21–30 minutes of medical discussion

On-Line Medical Evaluation

99444—For an established patient, guardian, or healthcare provider; may not have originated from a related E/M service provided within the previous 7 days.

Special Evaluation and Management Services

Medicare does not pay for these.

BASIC LIFE AND/OR DISABILITY EVALUATION SERVICES

99450—The four following elements are required:

- Measurement of height, weight, and blood pressure
- Completion of a medical history following a life insurance pro forma
- Collection of blood sample and/or urinalysis complying with "chain of custody" protocols
- Completion of necessary documentation/certificates

WORK-RELATED OR MEDICAL DISABILITY EVALUATION SERVICES

99455—Work-related medical disability examination done by the treating physician; the five following elements are required:

- Completion of medical history commensurate with the patient's condition
- Performance of an examination commensurate with the patient's condition
- Formulation of a diagnosis, assessment of capabilities and stability, and calculation of impairment
- Development of future medical treatment plan
- Completion of necessary documentation/certificates, and report

99456—Work-related medical disability examination done by provider other than the treating physician. Must include the same five elements listed for previous code.

This is just a partial list of codes found in the "Evaluation and Management" section of the CPT manual. We advise all psychiatrists and other mental health clinicians to purchase a copy of the manual to ensure access to information on the full range of codes.

QUESTIONS AND ANSWERS

Q. *Who may use E/M codes?*

A. Psychiatrists and appropriately licensed nurses and physician assistants may use the E/M codes.

Q. *Is a unit treatment team conference on an inpatient unit a service for which one may code?*

A. Treatment team conferences can be coded for but should be considered part of overall coordination of care. The time spent providing that service is a component of the total unit/floor time. Team conferences should not be coded as a separate service but rather as a component of the total services provided to the patient on any given day.

Q. *If I have a patient in the hospital whom I see for rounds in the morning and again when I am called to the ward in the afternoon because of a problem, do I code for two subsequent hospital care visits?*

A. No. One code should be selected that incorporates all of the hospital inpatient services provided that day.

Q. *What are the documentation requirements associated with inpatient and outpatient consultations?*

A. The request for the consultation must be documented in the patient's medical record. The consultant's opinion and any services that are performed also must be documented in the patient's medical record and communicated in writing to the requesting physician.

Q. *What codes should be used for psychiatric services provided in partial hospital settings, residential treatment facilities, and nursing homes?*

A. The codes for partial hospitalization services are the same as those used for hospital inpatient settings (99221–99239). The codes for residential treatment services are the same as those used for nursing facility services (99301–99316).

Q. *When would I use the pharmacological management code (90862) rather than one of the E/M outpatient codes?*

A. Your decision should be based on which code most accurately reports the services provided. Code 90862 is valued slightly less in relative value units than 99213, but 90862 is used specifically for psychopharmacological management. Code 99213 denotes more general medical services and might include consideration of comorbid medical conditions.

Q. *Is it necessary for the provider to record the examination him- or herself or can a checklist be used for the patient to record past history?*

A. A checklist is acceptable if the clinician provides a narrative report of the important positive and relevant negative findings. Abnormal findings should be described in the report. A notation of an abnormal finding without a description is not sufficient.

Q. *Can a checklist be used for an ROS?*

A. Yes, but pertinent positive and negative findings that are relevant to the presenting problem must be commented on by the examining clinician. Failure to document the appropriate number of systems for each level of service is the most common reason for downcoding by claims auditors, resulting in a lower level of reimbursement.

Q. *Now that Medicare no longer pays for consultation codes, how do I code for a consultation request from a colleague and what are the reporting requirements?*

A. When you are coding for Medicare or for commercial carriers that have followed Medicare's lead, 90801 may be used for both inpatient and outpatient consults. Psychiatrists who choose to use E/M codes to report outpatient consults should use the outpatient new patient codes (99201–99205). For inpatient consults, the codes to use are hospital inpatient services, initial hospital care for new or established patients (99221–99223). For consults in nursing homes, initial nursing facility care codes should be used (99304–99306); if the consult is of low complexity, the subsequent nursing facility codes may be used (99307–99310). As with all E/M codes, the selection of the specific code is based on the complexity of the case and the amount of work required. Medicare has created a new modifier, **A1,** to denote the admitting physician so that more than one physician may use the initial hospital care codes. It is still necessary to report back to the referring physician, but it is not necessary to write a report. The report can be done by telephone or the patient record can be sent to the referring physician.

Q. *Is it permissible to use a template or checklist to record the mental status examination?*

A. Yes.

Q. *If my mode of practice for inpatient services is to have an internist or family practitioner do a medical history and a physical examination and I then do the psychiatric evaluation and mental status examination within a 24-hour period, how can we code so we will both be paid?*

A. The typical way to code for this situation is to have the internist or family practitioner use a new patient E/M code and a medical diagnosis code and for the psychiatrist use a hospital service code for first day and a psychiatric diagnosis code.

5

Coding and Documentation for Specific Clinical Settings

This chapter provides suggested service codes for use in specific clinical settings and situations. Because there are choices to be made between evaluation and management (E/M) and psychiatric service codes in certain clinical circumstances, we provide alternative patterns of coding when appropriate. The reader is reminded to always use the code that best describes the service provided.

PRIVATE OFFICE AND OTHER OUTPATIENT FACILITIES

Initial Visit—Diagnostic Interview
- May be used by all appropriately licensed providers (M.D., R.N., Ph.D., L.C.S.W.).
- May require two or more sessions for geriatric or child/adolescent evaluation.
- May also be medically necessary based on major change in mental status.
- When the E/M codes for a new patient in an office or other outpatient setting (99201–99205) are being used, the documentation guidelines discussed in Chapter 4 must be followed.

Available codes	Average Medicare fees
90801	$153.72
90802	$165.27
99201	$38.97
99202	$67.48
99203	$97.79
99204	$151.56
99205	$190.53

Note.   Medicare fees are provided as a benchmark. The ones provided in this chapter are based on the 2010 Physician Fee Schedule. Medicare fees change almost every year and can be tracked by going to the Part B Fee Schedule for your local Medicare carrier or contractor.

Individual Psychotherapy

- Only psychiatrists and other duly licensed mental health providers may use the codes with E/M.
- Nonphysician therapists and psychiatrists may use codes without E/M.
- Codes are selected on the basis of time and whether E/M is included.

	Available codes	Average Medicare fees
With E/M	90805	$71.81
	90807	$100.68
	90809	$142.53
Without E/M	90804	$63.51
	90806	$88.05
	90808	$129.54

Pharmacological Management

- Physicians and other duly licensed prescribers.
- For Medicare, 90862 represents at least 15 minutes of face-to-face time with the patient, and Healthcare Common Procedure Coding System code M0064 represents 10 minutes of face-to-face time.
- When the E/M codes for an established patient in an office or other outpatient setting (99211–99213) are being used, the documentation guidelines discussed in Chapter 4 must be followed.

	Available codes	Average Medicare fees
	90862	$56.29
	M0064	$42.22
Return visit	99211	$19.12
	99212	$38.97
	99213	$65.67

Split Management of Outpatient Care Between Physician and Nonphysician Providers

INITIAL VISIT DIAGNOSTIC INTERVIEW

- Physicians and appropriately licensed nonphysicians.
- Medicare will usually accept only one 90801 for a new patient.

Available codes	Average Medicare fees
90801	$153.72
90802	$165.27

PHARMACOLOGICAL MANAGEMENT

- Physician only.

	Available codes	Average Medicare fees
	90862	$56.29
	M0064	$42.22
New patient	99201	$38.97
	99202	$67.48
Return visit	99211	$19.12
	99212	$38.97
	99213	$65.67

INDIVIDUAL PSYCHOTHERAPY WITHOUT EVALUATION AND MANAGEMENT

- Usually nonphysician.

Available codes	Average Medicare fees
90804	$63.51
90806	$88.05
90808	$129.54

OTHER PSYCHIATRIC SERVICES

	Available codes	Average Medicare fees
Psychoanalysis	90845	$81.91
Family psychotherapy without patient	90846	$86.60
Family psychotherapy with patient	90847	$107.89
Group psychotherapy	90853	$31.75

Office or Other Outpatient Evaluation and Management Services

These codes may be used only by physicians and other appropriately licensed providers. Some psychiatrists and nurse practitioners have outpatient practices focused on patients with major medical comorbidities who require a clinical emphasis on medical management rather than on psychotherapy. Under these clinical circumstances outpatient E/M codes may best represent the services provided to their patients.

> **Caution:** The documentation guidelines for E/M codes discussed in Chapter 4 must be followed when using these codes.

ESTABLISHED PATIENT—RETURN VISITS

	Available codes	Average Medicare fees
Five levels of service	99211	$19.12
	99212	$38.97
	99213	$65.67
	99214	$98.51
	99215	$132.79

OUTPATIENT OFFICE CONSULTATIONS

Note: Medicare no longer pays for these codes, and other insurers may follow suit. See discussion on alternative coding later in the chapter.

ACUTE HOSPITAL AND PARTIAL HOSPITAL SERVICES USING EVALUATION AND MANAGEMENT CODES

These services are provided *only* by attending psychiatrists. Most attending psychiatrists' care in hospitals or partial hospital programs is coded using E/M hospital service codes. However, Medicare and commercial insurers also permit use of certain 908xx codes to denote attending services. Both options are presented in the following sections.

Initial Hospital Care, New or Established Patient

- Because of the morbidity and complexity required for admission, most admission workups justify use of 99222 or 99223.
- Readmissions within 30 days are usually coded 99221 or 99222 because the data of the history have already been established. A higher-level code may be appropriate if the readmission is required because of a symptom change that requires complex medical decision making (e.g., a suicide attempt).

	Available codes	Average Medicare fees
Three levels of care	99221	$95.26
	99222	$129.18
	99223	$189.80
	or	
	90801	$153.72

Subsequent Hospital or Partial Hospital Care

- With lengths of stay averaging 6 days for most acute hospital admissions, the amount of attending work for subsequent care in the acute hospital setting justifies 99232, and on some days 99233.
- Partial hospital length of stay tends to be longer, and the appropriate codes are more likely to be 99231 and 99232.
- The attending psychiatrist will *not* be paid by Medicare for an inpatient psychotherapy code and a subsequent care E/M code on the same day. Another duly licensed clinician may provide individual psychotherapy, code for it, and be reimbursed.
- The attending psychiatrist may provide, code, and bill for group psychotherapy and subsequent hospital care on the same day.

	Available codes	Average Medicare fees
Three levels of care	99231	$38.25
	99232	$68.92
	99233	$98.87

Hospital Discharge Day

	Available codes	Average Medicare fees
Less than 30 minutes	99238	$67.84
More than 30 minutes	99239	$98.87

ALTERNATIVE CODING POSSIBILITIES FOR ADULT HOSPITAL AND PARTIAL HOSPITAL SERVICES

	Available codes	Average Medicare fees
Initial hospital care	90801	$127.38
	90802 (interactive)	$137.84
Daily subsequent care— medication management	90862	$45.47
Inpatient psychotherapy with E/M	90817	$66.40
	90819	$94.90
	90822	$136.76

> **Caution:** Use of the psychotherapy codes requires the attending to do face-to-face psychotherapy with the patient for the amount of time indicated by the code. The E/M component of these codes is less than 5 minutes of work.

Inpatient Consultation Services

Note: Medicare no longer pays for these codes, and other insurers may follow suit. See discussion on page 50 for alternative coding.

Follow-Up Care After Consultation

Follow-up consultation codes were eliminated from Current Procedural Terminology; instead use E/M subsequent care codes 99231–99233 (see page 50); medication management code 90862 (see page 19); or inpatient psychotherapy codes with E/M 90817, 90819, and 90822 (see page 16). Documentation guidelines for the 908xx and the E/M codes are discussed in Chapters 3 and 4, respectively.

EVALUATION AND MANAGEMENT NURSING FACILITY SERVICES

The following codes may also be used in psychiatric residential treatment centers.

Initial Nursing Facility Care, New or Established Patient

- These codes are used at the time of admission to a long-term care facility. Typically such a service is billed by the attending of record.

	Available codes	Average Medicare fees
Three levels of service	99304	$85.16
	99305	$119.44
	99306	$152.64

- If the psychiatrist is not the attending, a psychiatric diagnostic interview examination (90801; average Medicare fee: $147.02) may be used as the appropriate code for the service provided.
- Alternatively, if the psychiatrist is asked to perform a consult, he or she could code that visit using the nursing facility initial E/M codes. See Q&A on pages 60–61 for more information on coding for inpatient consults.

Subsequent Nursing Facility Care

If the psychiatrist is not the attending, care subsequent to a diagnostic evaluation (90801) or a consultation (99252–99255) may be as follows:

- Subsequent nursing facility care (99307–99310)
- Medication management (90862, average Medicare fee $45.08)
- Individual inpatient psychotherapy with E/M (90816/17, 90818/19, 90821/22, 90823/24, 90826/27, 90828/29)

	Available codes	Average Medicare fees
Four levels of care	99307	$40.78
	99308	$62.79
	99309	$82.99
	99310	$122.69

Caution: Psychotherapy provided to patients with dementia may be audited. The use of psychotherapy codes requires face-to-face time as noted for the code chosen. The E/M component is considered to be no more than 5 minutes of work.

Note: In nursing facilities, physicians sometimes get requests for second opinions that are not covered by Medicare. A second-opinion E/M service is a request from the patient and/or family or mandated (e.g., by a third-party payer) rather than from a physician or other qualified nonphysician provider. It is different from a consultation service requested by a physician, qualified nonphysician provider, or other appropriate source that meets the requirements for consultation services and should be reported using the initial hospital service codes. Medicare does not require that a written report be sent to a physician when a second-opinion evaluation has been requested by the patient and/or family. In fact, there is no average Medicare fee for a second-opinion evaluation because Medicare does not pay for this service. The service should be coded using 90899 (unlisted psychiatric service or procedure) or 99499 (unlisted evaluation or management service). When providing a second opinion, we recommend requesting an order from the physician of record.

6

Medicare

Medicare is a federal program that was established in 1965 as part of the Social Security Act to provide medical health benefits to people 65 and older and to people younger than 65 who qualify for Social Security Insurance because of a disability. The overall administration of Medicare is the purview of the Centers for Medicare and Medicaid Services (CMS).

Medicare is divided into three parts. Part A is essentially hospital insurance and covers expenses for care provided in a hospital, skilled nursing facility, nursing home, or hospice. It covers charges that are billed directly by the facility. Part A has been administered within each state by insurers who have been designated as *fiscal intermediaries*. Part B covers payments for professional services of physicians and nonphysician healthcare providers and a variety of outpatient services including X-rays, laboratory work, and durable medical equipment. Part B has been administered by insurers that serve as *Medicare carriers* in each state.

The Medicare program is currently in a period of transition. Changes are ongoing to consolidate the administration of Parts A and B under one contractor, a Medicare Administrative Contractor, and to have fewer contractors administrating Medicare over 15 jurisdictions, rather than state by state. (For a list of current contractors currently in place, see Appendix M.)

There are also Medicare Advantage plans, or managed Medicare plans, which cover both Part A and Part B and usually Part D (see below) for beneficiaries. These plans are sometimes referred to as Medicare + C or Medicare C. They are not really a separate part of the Medicare program, however, but just a way of accessing the other parts.

Since January 2006, there has also been Medicare Part D, the Medicare prescription drug benefit. This program is administered by private insurers overseen by CMS. Although clinicians often must navigate Part D to get their patients appropriate medications, they have no real relationship to Part D except when they assist with appeals for their patients.

Over the years since its inception the Medicare program has grown to become one of the largest payers of healthcare in the United States. You may ask why it is relevant to know about the Medicare program if your practice has few or no Medicare patients. The reason for understanding how the Medicare program works is that many elements of the program (including the Resource-Based Relative Value Scale [RBRVS] that is used for physician reimbursement) have been adopted by commercial carriers. Medicare tends to set the standard for how health insurance companies reimburse.

BASIC PAYMENT MECHANISM

Physician services provided on a fee-for-service basis (traditional Medicare, as opposed to Medicare Advantage, or Medicare provided through a health maintenance organization, other managed care organization, or private health plan) are paid as follows: Medicare patients must pay an annual deductible for Part B services (in 2010 it is $155), after which they have a copayment of 20% of the Medicare-allowed amount for most Part B services. For most outpatient psychiatric services, however, Medicare currently reimburses at 55% of the allowed amount for each service, leaving the patient (or the patient's secondary insurance) responsible for the other 45%. This is the result of something called the *outpatient mental health treatment limitation,* which Congress voted to phase out in the Medicare Improvements for Patients and Providers Act of 2008. The limitation is being phased out in stages (until 2010, Medicare paid only 50% rather than 55%) and will be totally eliminated as of 2014.

Every service covered under Medicare has a Medicare-allowed amount that can be billed for that service. Services not covered by Medicare are not reimbursed by the program and are the patient's responsibility, and the clinician may bill the patient whatever the standard office fee is for this service. (If a Current Procedural Terminology [CPT] code is not included on the physician fee schedule, which can be found on the contractor's Web site, that means that the code represents a noncovered service.) It is very important to document that the patient understands that the service is not covered under Medicare and still requests that it be provided. If the practitioner has reason to believe that a Medicare-covered service may not be considered medically necessary by Medicare, and hence will not be reimbursed by Medicare, the practitioner must issue the patient a document called an Advanced Beneficiary Notice if the patient is to be held responsible for the payment (see p. 79). For more information about this and other Medicare issues, you can contact the American Psychiatric Association (APA) Help Line at 800-343-4671.

PARTICIPATION AND NONPARTICIPATION

Practitioners who enroll to be Medicare providers have the option of being *participating* or *nonparticipating providers* (this is often shortened to *par* and *nonpar*). A *participating* provider accepts assignment, which means he or she is reimbursed directly by Medicare and the patient's out-of-pocket financial responsibility is limited to the copayment. A provider who is nonparticipating must still file the necessary forms with Medicare but collects the entire fee from the patient, who will then be reimbursed by Medicare. The advantage to being a nonparticipating provider is that you are permitted to charge a slightly higher fee than a participating provider. Each year every Medicare carrier posts the allowed fees for participating and nonparticipating providers on its Web site. Providers who do not have access to the Internet can contact their carrier (or contractor) by phone and request a hard copy of the fee schedule (see list of Medicare Carriers and Administrative Contractors in Appendix M for Web addresses and phone numbers).

To Participate or Not to Participate

If your practice includes even a moderate number of Medicare patients, participation may help your cash flow. Because 55%–80% (depending on the service provided) of the approved Medicare fee is paid directly to you rather than to the patient, your collection process probably will be faster, with fewer administrative hassles. In addition, you may have a decided competitive edge; patients may select you because they know your participation means they will only be responsible for the copayment for covered services.

The advantages of nonparticipation are that 1) you are able to accept assignment and function just like a participating provider on a claim-by-claim basis, giving you freedom of choice, which may be philosophically important to you (although as a nonpar provider you can bill for only 95% of the allowed amount); and 2) you are allowed to bill patients for covered services at 15% above the Medicare-allowed amount (balance billing) when you do not participate. Offsetting that billing advantage is the fact that Medicare payments for nonparticipating physicians are 95% of the payment rates for participating physicians, which effectively reduces the 15% additional billing amount to 9.25%. Clinical psychologists and social workers are obligated to accept assignments, so they would have nothing to gain by choosing to be nonpar.

MEDICARE PHYSICIAN PAYMENT REFORM

The current Medicare physician payment system, which went into effect on January 1, 1992, was the result of a decade of joint effort by the federal government and the medical profession to alter the way Medicare paid for physician services (this covers all provider payments, not just payments to physicians). Prior to this, all physician payments had been based on a system of customary, prevailing, and reasonable charges, although Medicare had placed a series of controls on reimbursement levels that essentially held reimbursement to early 1970s levels.

Even though there was widespread dissatisfaction with the level of reimbursement, no substitute method for payment was considered acceptable until the development of the RBRVS. In addition, the government wanted to bring its Part B payment system in line with its Part A payment system, which in 1983 became largely a prospective payment system, using diagnosis-related groups (DRGs) as the basis for reimbursing hospitals. The first relative value scale was created by the California Medical Association in 1956, based on median charges reported by California Blue Shield. This system of payment was eventually used by a number of state Medicaid programs, Blue Cross/Blue Shield plans, and several other commercial insurers to set fee schedules. During the late 1970s, however, the Federal Trade Commission raised concerns about the possibility of antitrust violations, and the California Medical Association suspended the use of its relative value scale.

Under pressure to come up with an alternative payment system for physician services, the Health Care Financing Administration (HCFA; now CMS) turned to a research team at the Harvard School of Public Health led by Drs. William Hsaio, a health economist, and Peter Braun, a physician. Their work resulted in the development of the RBRVS for physician payment, which was adopted by HCFA and the Physician Payment Review Commission of Congress and implemented in 1992. The RBRVS calculates the work required for each service covered by Medicare in relative value units, or RVUs, which are also used to account for practice and medical liability expenses. The creation of the RBRVS was supported by the American Medical Association (AMA). In cooperating with HCFA on the development of the RBRVS, the AMA insisted on the following features that became part of the system:

- Payment schedule amounts should be adjusted to reflect geographic differences in physicians' practice costs, such as office rent and wages of nonphysician personnel.
- Geographic differences in the cost of physicians' professional liability insurance would be especially important, and these differences should be reflected separately from other practice costs.
- There should be a transition period in the implementation of the system to minimize disruption in patient care and access.
- Organized medicine would seek to play a major role in updating the RBRVS.

The new payment reform affected all physician services. The only exceptions were physician services provided to Medicare patients enrolled in Medicare health maintenance organizations and certain services provided by teaching physicians in hospitals, skilled nursing facilities, and comprehensive outpatient rehabilitation facilities. Since 1998, services provided by nonphysician providers (Ph.D.'s, social workers, and others) are also covered by the RBRVS.

The AMA publishes *Medicare RBRVS: The Physicians' Guide,* which is updated every year. The book is divided into five sections: "Roots of Medicare's RBRVS Payment System," "Major Components of the RBRVS Payment System," "RBRVS Payment System and Operation," "RBRVS Payment System in Your Practice," and reference lists and appendixes. It contains valuable information about the RBRVS that can be applied directly to your practice. The book can be ordered by writing the Medicare RBRVS Order Department, OP059698, American Medical Association, 515 North State Street, Chicago, Illinois, 60610, or by calling 800-621-8335.

COMPUTING MEDICARE FEES

Medicare fees are established by the U.S. Congress through an update process that was modified as part of the Balanced Budget Act of 1997 and again by the Balanced Budget Refinement Act of 1999. Using a construct called the Sustainable Growth Rate (SGR), a conversion factor is computed for each fiscal year. The Medicare allowable fee for any medical service is computed each year by multiplying the total RVUs that have been assigned to that service by the year's conversion factor.

EXAMPLE OF COMPUTATION OF FEES FOR 90801 IN 2010			
90801 Psychiatric diagnostic interview examination (non-facility)			
Work relative value unit (RVU)	Practice expense RVUs	Professional liability RVUs	Total RVUs
2.80	1.38	0.08	4.26
RVUs x 2010 conversion factor = 2010 fee for 90801 2010 conversion factor = $36.0864 4.26 x $36.0864 = **$153.73**			

The range of RVUs, and therefore the fees for mental health services (90800 series and evaluation and management [E/M] 99000 series) is narrow compared with the RVUs for other medical services.

RANGE OF RELATIVE VALUE UNITS (RVUs) AND FEES FOR MENTAL HEALTH PROFESSIONALS	
Psychiatric codes	90800 series (non-facility)
RVUs	0.88 (90853) to 4.58 (90802)
Fees	$31.75 to $165.27
Evaluation and management codes	99000 series (non-facility)
RVUs	0.53 (99211) to 6.28 (99245)
Fees	$19.12 to $226.61

MEDICARE PAYMENT POLICIES

Telephone Management

Payment is not made for telephone consultations. CMS considers this part of pre- or postservice work, which is calculated into the work RVUs.

Injections

If you provide a subcutaneous intramuscular or intravenous injection in conjunction with a patient visit, no additional payment is made for administering the injection. However, separate payment is made for the drug injected. CMS considers the resource costs of administering the drug (including nondrug supplies) to be bundled into the payment for the visit.

Nonphysicians and Medicare

The Medicare program provides payment for clinical psychologists, clinical social workers, physician assistants, nurse-practitioners, and clinical nurse specialists. All of these clinicians must be licensed in their states to perform the services they provide.

- **Clinical psychologists**—As of January 1, 1997, Medicare payment for diagnostic and therapeutic services provided by clinical psychologists was incorporated into the RBRVS and is paid at 100% of the Medicare RBRVS amount. Outpatient services other than diagnostic services have been subject to the outpatient mental health services limitation, which will be eliminated in 2014, just as when these services are provided by physicians.
- **Clinical social workers (CSWs)**—CSWs are paid at 75% of the payment schedule amount, or the Medicare RBRVS amount, for the therapeutic services they provide. For diagnostic services CSWs are paid at the same rate as physicians and clinical psychologists.
- **Physician assistants (PAs)**—Since the passage of the Balanced Budget Act of 1997, states have been permitted to determine the required level of physician supervision for PAs. Most states permit the physician to be available to the assistant by electronic means rather than having to be in the same space. Physician assistants may be employed by physicians or may be independent contractors. Payment is 85% of the Medicare-allowed amount for the service or the actual charge, whichever is lower.
- **Nurse-practitioners (NPs) and clinical nurse specialists (CNSs)**—Since 1997, NPs and CNSs have been permitted to practice without direct physician supervision. They can be paid directly by Medicare and are paid 85% of the Medicare allowed amount or the actual charge, whichever is lower.

"Incident to" Services

Incident to services must be provided under the direct supervision of a physician or other authorized practitioner. This means the supervisor must be "*present in the office suite and immediately available to provide assistance and direction throughout the time the aide is performing services*." Incident to services are billed under the physician's name.

In 2002, new regulations covering billing for incident to services went into effect. They state that Medicare pays for services provided by auxiliary personnel that are incident to physician services without regard to the employment relationship of the aide either to the physician or to the entity that employs the aide.

Medicare Teaching-Physician Rules

On December 8, 1995, HCFA issued new regulations revising the rules for Medicare Part B payment for services of teaching physicians. The new regulations became effective July 1, 1996.

General rule. If a resident (or fellow) participates in a service furnished in a teaching setting, a Part B payment will be allowed only if the teaching physician is present during the key portion of any service or procedure for which payment is sought. An attending physician relationship is no longer required in order to code and bill, and the term *attending physician* was replaced with *teaching physician.* Each physician will determine the key portion of any service or procedure furnished. This concept is intended to provide flexibility to the rule and to avoid requiring the presence of the teaching physician for the full duration of every service or procedure coded and billed in his or her name. Although CMS understands that it may be difficult for providers to determine the key portion for every particular service, the concept is necessarily general because it is not feasible to define the key portion for all services prospectively.

These rules are necessary because teaching hospitals are paid at a higher rate by Medicare than nonteaching hospitals to take into account the presence of residents and fellows who will be participating in the facility care provided by the hospital.

CMS established an exception for services provided by psychiatric residents. This exception permits the physical presence requirement for the teaching physician to be met via one-way mirrors or video equipment as long as the teaching physician meets with the patient following the visit.

The Correct Coding Initiative and Medically Unlikely Edits

Because CMS pays the majority of Medicare claims as submitted, over the years CMS has sought to find ways to ensure that only valid claims are paid, rather than picking up errors using postpayment reviews. Currently there are two programs that attempt to do this: the Correct Coding Initiative and Medically Unlikely Edits.

The Correct Coding Initiative (CCI) is a lengthy list of Current Procedural Codes (CPT) codes that cannot be filed on the same day by the same provider, often because the service provided by one code is supposed to be included in the other. For psychiatric services, it forbids using an E/M code and one of the psychotherapy codes with E/M (90805, 90807, 90809) on the same day. The reason is that these psychotherapy codes already include evaluation and management. Some of the edits can be overridden by using a CPT modifier.

Medically Unlikely Edits (MUEs) were first used in 2007 to delineate services that were essentially medically impossible for anatomical reasons. For instance, eye surgery could not be done on more than two eyes; a left thumb could only be amputated once; and a hysterectomy could not be done on a male patient. More edits are expected to be added in the future, some of which may have an impact on mental health services by limiting the number of encounters a provider may have with a patient on one day.

Medicare as Secondary Payer

When a patient has Medicare but is still employed, or is the spouse of someone who is still employed, Medicare will be the secondary payer. If the amount the primary payer allows for the service is higher than what Medicare allows, Medicare will pay the amount up to the higher fee to a participating provider (as long as the amount paid by Medicare does not exceed the Medicare-allowed amount). For instance, if the employer insurance allows $150 for a service but pays only 80% of that amount, or $120, even though the Medicare-allowed amount for that service is $125, Medicare will pay $30 so the physician will be fully reimbursed at the primary insurer's rate. However, *nonparticipating providers whose patients pay up front may only have the patient pay up to the Medicare limiting amount, no matter what the primary insurer pays.* To learn all the details about Medicare as secondary payer from the beneficiary's point of view, you can download a booklet on the topic at http://www.medicare.gov/Publications/Pubs/pdf/02179.pdf.

WHAT IS AN LCD?

An LCD (local coverage determination) represents a decision by a Medicare contractor (either Part A, Part B, or both) as to whether a service is reasonable and necessary and hence will be paid for by Medicare.

LCDs may provide the following criteria and guidelines:

- The general indications for which a service is covered or considered medically necessary.
- The ICD codes (diagnostic codes) or code ranges for which the service is generally covered and/or considered medically necessary.
- The clinicians who may provide the service.
- Diagnoses that support medical necessity.
- Limitations or situations in which the service would not be considered medically necessary.
- ICD codes (diagnostic codes) that do not support medical necessity of the service (this may just be any codes that were not listed as covered).
- Specific situations under which the service will always be denied, with a list of the reasons for the denial.
- Noncovered ICD codes (diagnostic codes)—that is, medical diagnoses for which the service will always be denied.
- Coding guidelines, including information about units of service, place of service, and modifiers.
- Documentation requirements—that is, specific information from medical records or other information that would be required to justify the service.
- Information concerning the typical or expected utilization for the service.

Medical reviewers for carriers and fiscal intermediaries use the information provided in LCDs to decide whether claims for treatment are paid or denied. As noted, LCDs often delineate which diagnoses will be covered for which CPT codes and what kind of documentation is needed to support specific codes. They may also indicate how many treatments are permitted over a certain length of time.

Carriers must present new LCDs to their Carrier Advisory Committees, which comprise representatives from local medical specialty groups, for discussion and approval. Carriers and fiscal intermediaries are also required to have open meetings so that interested members of the public can provide comments on draft LCDs. In recent years, as the psychiatry LCDs have come up for modification, the psychiatry representatives to the Carrier Advisory Committees, working with American Psychiatric Association (APA) district branches and the APA's Office of Healthcare Systems and Financing, have been very active in working to ensure that the revised LCDs accurately reflect psychiatry as it is currently practiced.

Currently all draft and final LCDs must be posted on the Internet. They can be accessed on your Medicare contractor's Web site (see Appendix M) or on the CMS Web site by going to www.cms.hhs.gov/mcd/search.asp.

ADVANCE BENEFICIARY NOTICE

If you provide a service that you think Medicare *may not* reimburse for, because Medicare may not deem it medically necessary or for any other reason, you must issue your patient an Advance Beneficiary Notice before you perform the service or the patient will have no legal obligation to pay for the Medicare-rejected service out of pocket. A copy of the newly revised notice can be accessed on the CMS website at http://www.cms.hhs.gov/BNI/02_ABN.asp.

OPTING OUT OF MEDICARE AND PRIVATE CONTRACTING

Physicians and other practitioners are permitted to have private contracts with Medicare patients for healthcare services, provided they opt out of Medicare entirely by filing an opt-out affidavit with their Medicare carrier (or Medicare Administrative Contractor). A practitioner opts out for a period of 2 years (which can be renewed at the end of that time for as long as the provider wants to continue practicing outside the Medicare program). During those 2 years, the clinician may not see any patients under Medicare. This means that if patients with Medicare coverage receive services from a practitioner who has opted out, they will not be able to receive any reimbursement from Medicare. For this reason, clinicians who opt out of Medicare must have each of their Medicare patients fill out a private contract that documents that Medicare cannot be billed for any services performed by the clinician and that the patient understands this.

The advantage to opting out is that you can charge your standard fees rather than only being permitted to bill the Medicare-allowed amount. The disadvantages are that many patients will not be able to afford to see you and that if you should change your practice situation during your 2-year opt-out period and need to see Medicare patients as part of your new work, you will not be able to do so.

More information about opting out of Medicare is available to members on the APA's Web site (www.psych.org) or you can call the APA Managed Care Help Line at 800-343-4671.

MEDICARE ADVANTAGE

More than 6 million Medicare beneficiaries are now enrolled in Medicare Advantage managed care plans, including so-called private fee-for-service plans, which supposedly allow enrollees to see any physician they choose. If your patient is enrolled in a Medicare Advantage plan from a network that you participate in, you will be paid the amount for the service specified in your contract for the service you provide. If you do not participate in the plan's network, the plan is obligated to pay you the same amount you would receive for the service from the Medicare Part B carrier.

QUESTIONS AND ANSWERS

Q. *I'm not taking any more Medicare patients. A man with Medicare coverage has said he would like me to be his therapist and would be willing to pay out of pocket because I am not accepting anymore Medicare patients. Can I see him as a non-Medicare patient?*

A. The simple answer is no. The only time a Medicare patient can be seen outside Medicare is if the patient requests this because of a desire that originates with the patient (not as a response to the provider's unwillingness to bill Medicare).

Q. *It is our office policy to charge patients for missed appointments. I know that Medicare does not cover this. Does this mean we cannot bill our Medicare patients for missed appointments?*

A. No, it does not mean that. Because charges for missed appointments are absolutely not paid for by Medicare, you are free to charge your Medicare patients the standard office fee for missing an appointment. However, you must be sure that you have documentation that the patient was informed of this policy and that the same policy applies to all of your patients.

Q. *If I am a nonparticipating provider (I do not accept Medicare assignment), can I charge a Medicare patient my full standard fee for a covered service?*

A. Nonparticipating providers are allowed to bill Medicare patients for covered services slightly above the Medicare-approved amount. There is a limiting charge for nonparticipating providers, which is set at 15% above the Medicare-approved amount for participating providers. Because Medicare-approved amounts for nonparticipating providers are 95% of the amounts for participating providers, this means you actually receive only 9.25% more reimbursement than you would as a participating provider.

Q. *Are there limiting charges for services not covered by Medicare?*

A. As noted in the answer to Question 2, if a service is not covered by Medicare you are free to charge your usual and customary fee to Medicare beneficiaries because there is no Medicare-allowed amount for that particular service. However, you must be sure your patient understands the service is not covered by Medicare and agrees to pay out of pocket for it if you wish to be reimbursed for providing it.

Q. *Can I waive the deductible or copayment for an indigent patient covered by Medicare?*

A. No. You are required by law to make a good faith effort to collect copayments and deductibles from all your patients. This means you must be able to show that you have sent bills, made telephone calls, and so on in an effort to collect what you are owed. Under the RBRVS provider payment system, if copayments and/or deductibles are routinely waived, the charge minus the copayment or deductible portion of the fee would be considered to be the actual charge for the service and thus Medicare would only be required to reimburse 80%, or 55%, of that smaller amount.

Q. *I see very few Medicare patients. Is there any reason for me to study and understand the RBRVS Medicare system of payment to providers?*

A. The Medicare RBRVS payment system is now being used by many commercial carriers. Therefore, it makes sense for you to become familiar with this payment system even if your contact with Medicare is limited.

Q. *I have been asked by the attorney for the family of a Medicare beneficiary to do a psychiatric evaluation of the beneficiary to attempt to determine his competence to make decisions. Am I bound by the Medicare fee schedule for the evaluation?*

A. Because the evaluation is not being done for the benefit of the Medicare beneficiary to determine treatment but rather for the family, it is not a covered procedure under Medicare and therefore you are not bound by the Medicare fee schedule. You would do well to explain this in writing to the person who will be paying for the evaluation.

Q. *I am going into private practice and want to opt out of Medicare, but I also will be working at a research facility where we see some Medicare patients. No fees are charged for services at the research facility. Can I opt out of Medicare and still see patients there who have Medicare?*

A. Yes, you can opt out of Medicare as long as Medicare will not be billed for any of the services you provide.

7

Commercial Insurance Issues

ROLE OF PRIVATE HEALTH INSURANCE COMPANIES IN THE MEDICAL SYSTEM

In the United States today private health insurance is generally employer sponsored. According to the Kaiser Family Foundation, in 2008 almost 158 million nonelderly people received their health insurance through employers, while another more than 13 million bought their health insurance directly from commercial insurers. Since 1965 the elderly and disabled have had their healthcare covered by Medicare, and the Medicaid program has provided healthcare for the poor.

CHANGES IN THE HEALTHCARE SYSTEM

After World War II, when employer-based health insurance first became the norm, most plans were indemnity plans, with employees seeing their healthcare providers just as they had done before, and the providers being paid their usual and customary fees, only now they were paid by the insurer rather than the patient. At that time there were a few prepaid group practice plans on the East and West Coasts, the prototypes for today's health maintenance organizations (HMOs), that were apparently providing cost-effective and quality care, but the number of people they covered was not significant. (It should be noted that although the American Medical Association fought their existence throughout the 1930s and 1940s, by the 1950s it had come to accept their small presence in the healthcare universe.)

It could be said that the current world of managed care began when Richard Nixon signed the HMO Act of 1973 into law and the federal government began providing funds to encourage the growth of HMOs. Believe it or not, it was the hope of the Nixon administration that healthcare in the United States would all be covered by HMOs like the one that Kaiser ran so successfully in President Nixon's home state of California. Over time it became clear that existing HMOs such as Kaiser would not expand to absorb the entire population of the United

States, nor was there much incentive for new organizations to pick up the slack, because the existing HMOs were all nonprofits. However, the seeds for delivering healthcare in a new way had been planted.

By the late 1980s, as employers were finding fee-for-service health insurance more and more expensive to sustain, a variety of managed care plans began to emerge that offered them lower-cost care while still providing their employees with comprehensive coverage. The expectation was that a focus on health maintenance and the replacement of fee-for-service reimbursement (a cost-plus reimbursement model) with capitation (a risk reimbursement model) would control healthcare costs. The resulting HMO and managed care organization (MCO) models and insurance products did seem to lower costs for a while. However, the savings went mostly to private companies and their stockholders—not back into healthcare. Private entrepreneurs leapt at the opportunity to make profits by limiting access to care for patients and shifting the risk of costs to physicians and other providers. The impact of this on mental health services has been especially difficult for patients and providers alike.

However, when it comes to deciding about access to care and documentation of services, the HMO/MCO requirements are actually simplified. If reimbursement is based on capitation, utilization of services is the provider's issue, as are coding and documentation. If, on the other hand, reimbursement is by a contracted fee schedule, the HMO is concerned principally about utilization, which it controls through pre-established fees, allowed services, preset numbers of services, authorization for services, and periodic justification for recurring services (e.g., psychotherapy). Some MCOs carve out the behavioral health benefit to a managed behavioral health organization, which manages the mental health benefits and fees just like any other MCO.

The problems for practitioners who contract with HMOs/MCOs usually involve fighting on behalf of their patients for access to care. Coding and documentation rarely are issues. The reverse situation pertains to Medicare, Medicaid, and indemnity programs.

With the vast majority of patients now insured through managed care, it is difficult for most practitioners to avoid contracting with MCOs, even though it may mean lower fees. Concurrent with the shift to managed care, and in part related to it, the health provider's work life has become a nightmare of paperwork. Each contract with each MCO is different. Some may permit only certain CPT codes to be billed by mental health providers; each has a different procedure for authorizing care. The problems created may prove especially daunting for those in solo or small group practices.

The negative impact of changes in the practice environment is pervasive. Patients are upset with providers' and health insurance companies' increased costs. Insurance companies complain that patients overuse services and accuse providers of inflating charges. Clinicians are wary of patients who demand high-quality care at discounted fees and yet are ready to pounce on any medical outcome that is less than perfect. The relationship between providers and health insurance companies is strained because cost management techniques have intruded into clinician decision making. It is within the context of this environment that you must manage the business aspects of your practice.

ORGANIZATION

Insurance companies are generally large for-profit organizations with many levels of management. Most companies employ physicians in a variety of positions, including that of medical director, and most companies have a medical advisory board composed of community physicians who serve voluntarily. Non-physician medical representatives are usually employed to help service relationships with physician providers. Despite the layers of management, which include physicians and specific programs for provider relations, practitioners often have difficulty accessing the decision-making apparatus of health insurance organizations.

CLAIMS MANAGEMENT AND REVIEW

One of the most important activities performed by insurance companies is processing claims and reimbursing providers of health services. That being the case, you would expect this activity to be a high priority for insurance companies. However, claims processing remains a relatively low-tech, trouble-plagued operation and causes more problems and frustration for patients, physicians, and the companies themselves than any other aspect of their business operations. The development of ever-more-sophisticated information systems and databases has improved the situation to some degree, but these changes have also created some new problems.

For providers who still file paper claims, the processing usually begins in the mailroom of the insurance company, where attachments to a claim are removed along with staples and paper clips in preparation for processing. The claim then goes to the claims processors, who are typically recent high-school graduates paid minimum wage. These initial processors usually are not trained in medical terminology or coding. Their task is to sort the claims and enter them into the computer or return the claims because they are incomplete. Claims that are returned include those with missing diagnoses, dates of service, or signatures. The claims processors are required to process a certain number of claims within a given time period, whether the claims are entered or returned. A claim returned for missing data takes a fraction of the time required to enter a processed claim. When pressed for time, processors will sometimes return claims for more information because that task is easier than processing the claim. The potential pitfalls of claims processing constitute one good reason for submitting claims electronically rather than manually, because the claims processor is bypassed.

Once entered into the computer system, the claim is reviewed by a claims examiner, who also typically has only a high-school education, is paid a relatively low wage, and has had limited training in medical terminology and coding. If the examiner understands the claim and agrees with the medical necessity for the service or procedure, payment will be authorized. However, if the examiner does not understand what was done for the patient and why it was done, the examiner may take one of three actions: 1) return the claim for more information; 2) refer the claim for review at a higher technical level (nurse or physician review);

or 3) file the claim for later review, which often leads to a delayed decision or disappearance of the claim altogether.

Clearly, problems for your claim can occur anywhere within the process. Your claims forms should always be filled out completely and legibly. Strategies to protect your claim are discussed in Chapter 8.

OVERSIGHT

Insurance companies are regulated in each state by the office of the insurance commissioner. The responsibility of the commissioner is to ensure that companies comply with state laws, maintain sufficient reserves, and conduct yearly audits. If you have reason to believe that an insurance company is operating in a way that does not comply with the law, you should contact the office of the insurance commissioner.

In addition to being subject to the oversight of the insurance commissioner, the public service role of insurance companies often attracts the attention of state legislators. The companies in turn employ lobbyists to influence the development of legislation beneficial to their operations. For the most part, their lobbying efforts are effective and balance the controls of the state insurance commissioner.

STRATEGIES FOR DEALING WITH INSURANCE COMPANIES

If you can understand the goals of the insurers, their priorities, their function within the health care system, and their organization, you are well on your way to developing effective strategies for dealing with them.

Developing and Maintaining Relationships With Insurance Companies

1. *Maintain businesslike, cordial relationships with the insurance company and its personnel.* No matter how frustrated you may become, always remember the company has many ways of retaliating. It can slow down processing of your claims, slow down reimbursement, and, most troublesome of all, audit you.
2. *Do not be intimidated by the insurance company.* Your relationship with the insurance company is strictly business, and there are rules and regulations that it must obey. The state insurance commissioner, the Better Business Bureau, the local medical society, your local professional society, and your legislators may be useful resources in selected incidents or disputes with a health insurance company (see "When Things Go Wrong" later in this chapter).
3. *Remember that an insurance company's first priority should be its customer—your patient.* Both you and the insurance company are providing a service to your patient. Within the boundaries of concerns about transference-countertransference issues, keep your patient informed about both good and bad aspects of your business relationship with the insurance company and health plan. The feedback you provide the patient may affect his or her own interactions with the company.

4. *Develop and maintain contact with one or two employees in each insurance company.* You or your office manager should foster friendly relationships with people in each insurance company with which you deal. If you succeed in developing such relationships, you will have people inside the companies who know you and can help solve problems.

5. *Consider filing a record of your mode of practice with the insurance company.* Many group practices place on record with carriers information about their mode of practice, including the services they intend to provide, any unusual features of their practice (e.g., group rather than solo coverage of inpatient services), the codes to be used for reporting, a list of the individual providers, and the fees they intend to charge. The benefits of placing this information on record with the carrier are that 1) problems with the mode of practice can be identified in advance and dealt with prospectively, 2) the record is a baseline set of data that helps the company make adjustments when any aspect of practice is changed, 3) the recorded mode also may serve as protection when disputes are caused by changes in company policies or operations that are not communicated to the provider, and 4) the record may serve as a protection when disputes trigger audits. The best person to contact in the insurance company to record your mode of practice or changes in your mode is the medical director of the company. The second choice for contact is the staff in the medical policy division.

6. *Document all contacts with insurance companies.* Keep all written materials that pass between you and insurance companies on file. Whenever you contact a company by telephone, record the name of the person with whom you spoke, that person's telephone number, and the date of the contact. As a follow-up to the telephone contact, send a memo to that person with a short, clear synopsis of the content of the call. If certain verbal agreements were made, document those agreements.

7. *Stay informed about the insurance companies with whom you do business.* Most companies periodically publish newsletters or directives to providers; read them carefully. Local and national newspapers regularly carry stories about insurance companies; although they may make for dry reading, the stories could contain useful information. Other sources of information about insurance companies and their operations and products are your local specialty society and the local medical society.

When Things Go Wrong

The likelihood that you will someday have a significant dispute with an insurance company is high. Because every claim represents a portion of your revenue stream, you must follow up assertively on all returned or rejected claims.

1. *Always remember this when dealing with an insurance company: It is business—not personal.* You are dealing with a large, impersonal bureaucracy that has many resources and means of retaliation. Keep your contacts businesslike and cordial.

2. *Be persistent in your efforts to resolve any disputes.* Only you can decide how much effort should be expended in resolving any given dispute. Remem-

ber, however, that repeated, businesslike contacts will eventually gain you access to an individual who can make decisions and help you.

3. *Enlist the help of your patient.* Remember that your patient is the insurance company's customer and its first priority. If you are making no progress, ask the patient to inquire about the disputed claim(s). The patient's request may be addressed while yours continues to be shuffled about. A patient's request for review of a claim usually requires some paperwork. It is in your best interest to help the patient complete the required paperwork. Information about health plan benefits and the mechanics of resolving disputed claims also may be available from the employee's company benefits manager (usually in the human resources department).

4. *Determine if there are any mechanisms for appeal.* If you cannot resolve an issue, ask the insurance company or insurance plan for the details of the formal appeals process.

5. *Look for help.* The following are some options:

   - *Peers*—Your colleagues are an important source of information about insurance problems. Describe your problem to physician friends; they may have had similar problems, and their experiences may provide answers for you. If the problem is shared by other physicians, consider a presentation to the insurance committee of your local specialty society.

   - *Local professional society*—Most local professional societies have standing insurance committees or committees on third-party relationships. These committees act as a clearinghouse for members who have problems with insurance companies. The knowledge and experience of the committees are often helpful to members who have disputes with insurance carriers. (The local medical society also may be helpful.) If your local professional society is unable to assist you, it can turn to the parent organization.

   - *Legal counsel*—From time to time there will be disputes with insurance companies that require the use of legal counsel. The cost of legal expertise is usually prohibitive for the practitioner, but if colleagues are experiencing the same problem, the shared cost may be affordable. The best way to determine the impact of your problem on your peers is through your local professional society. The society may even organize and financially support a legal strategy to solve a problem.

   - *Insurance commissioner*—If you believe your problem with a company represents a significant breach of the regulations governing the operation of insurance companies in your state, you can request the commissioner's review. This review is serious business, and such requests should not be made in anger or frivolously.

Again, if you use any or all of these suggestions, remember that your dispute with a company is a business issue—no matter how personally that issue affects you. Be cordial but determined. If you encounter a problem that seems unsolvable, call your professional organization. American Psychiatric Association members can receive help from the Managed Care Help Line at 800-343-4671 or hsf@psych.org. (See Appendix L for contact information for other clinicians.)

QUESTIONS AND ANSWERS

Q. *How can I protect my paper claims from being returned to me for what seem to be minor reasons?*

A. Fill out the forms completely and legibly. Stamp or write on attachments "Please do not separate attachments."

Q. *How can my local professional society help me when I have problems with an insurance company?*

A. Your local professional society can help in several ways. It can

- Put you in touch with colleagues who have similar problems
- Work with the insurance company to resolve the problem on behalf of you and other members
- Assist you in gaining access to association resources
- Sponsor legislation
- Organize and sponsor legal actions

Q. *Is it ethical to tell patients about problems I am having with their insurance companies?*

A. Informing patients about your problems with their insurance companies is not unethical. In fact, asking patients for their assistance in resolving a disputed claim by suggesting that they request a review of the claim can be a helpful tactic.

Q. *Can I realistically expect to challenge one of these big companies over any issue?*

A. A single practitioner will have difficulty influencing a company. By joining together with colleagues and enlisting the aid of your local professional society, you gain the strength of group action, which may succeed where your individual effort would not.

Q. *How can HMOs or managed care companies restrict physicians' access to certain service codes?*

A. The CPT manual and its codes are conventions for reporting and recording services. Insurance and managed care companies may specify which service codes physicians can and cannot use in the contracts you sign with them.

8

Putting It All Together for Accurate Coding

By the time you have reached this chapter, it should be completely clear that accurate coding and appropriate documentation are essential for supporting the billing and collection functions of your practice. The universal use of Current Procedural Terminology (CPT) codes for procedures and the ICD codes for diagnoses mandated by the Health Insurance Portability and Accountability Act (HIPAA), paired with readily available information technology, allows health insurers and the federal government (Centers for Medicare and Medicaid Services) to create databases of physicians' billing activity that can be easily retrieved and analyzed in many different ways. (See Appendix B for details about HIPAA and changes that will be coming.) These databases are being used to monitor and audit practices to achieve the payer's goal of efficient utilization of treatment resources.

Information technologies are a permanent part of the medical landscape, and there is a serious movement in the political world to have them become more and more pervasive, driven by evidence that they can make healthcare delivery more efficient and more effective. (Medicare has recently undertaken an incentive program to move clinicians into using electronic medical records (EMRs) and in 2015 will have in place a payment system that will penalize providers who have not converted.)

Clinicians must learn to use the products of technology constructively to improve patient care and also to protect the financial basis of their practices. The bottom-line message is that the business aspects of your practice must be absolutely shipshape if you want to ensure that you are appropriately reimbursed for your services in a timely manner. Coding needs to be accurate. Time spent resubmitting claims or resolving claim disputes results in lost time and dollars. Do it right the first time.

This chapter provides a practical guide to coding and documentation that should assist you in filing claims accurately and efficiently.

STEP 1: IDENTIFY AND RECORD EVERY SERVICE YOU PROVIDE

You are probably proficient in documenting the services you perform most frequently, such as new patient evaluations, psychotherapy sessions, and hospital visits. The fewer kinds of services and procedures you provide patients, the easier it is to track and record those services and procedures. For example, recording the services in an office practice with patients scheduled for psychotherapy *x* number of hours per day and *y* number of days per week is a straightforward process. However, many psychiatric practices offer complex, multiple services at various sites (e.g., in the office, hospital, partial hospitalization program, emergency department), with varying levels and times of service. If you wait until the end of the day and rely on your memory to tally up all of the services you provided at the various service sites, you can easily forget some billable services. To save time, make a checklist with the services, codes, diagnoses, and locations you use most frequently. Keep copies of the list in a notebook or on your laptop and record every service immediately after the service is provided.

It is possible that you provide some services to patients every day that you have never thought of as being worthy of being recorded for eventual billing (e.g., making telephone calls, writing reports and letters, providing educational supplies and patient information, incurring unusual travel costs). With the persistent, downward pressure on provider reimbursement, you may want to consider charging for some of these services. If you do this, you must discipline yourself to record them as systematically as you record the more commonly provided services that you already bill for. Of course, before you start charging for anything new, you must inform your patients that you will be charging for previously free services, because it is likely that most of them will not be paid for by insurers and the patients will have to pay for them out of pocket. Remember, for services that are specifically *not* covered under Medicare, Medicare patients can be asked to pay the standard office fee out of pocket, but you must be sure to document that when they began treatment with you they understood that they would be expected to pay this fee.

STEP 2: SELECT A CODE

The basic principle in selecting a CPT code is: *Select the code that most accurately reflects the service or procedure you provided to your patient.*

If your practice is office based and your services consist mostly of psychiatric evaluation and therapeutic procedures, you will be using codes 90801–90899, and you should have no problems matching procedures to codes.

Codes 90882–90899 cover a variety of services: environmental intervention for medical management, evaluation of hospital records, interpretation of results, preparation of reports, and unlisted services. These services are increasingly important in the era of managed care and accurately reflect much of the non-face-to-face work that must be done on the patient's behalf. However, Medicare and an increasing number of commercial insurers will not reimburse for these services. Nevertheless, when these services are provided distinct from the evaluation and management (E/M) services provided in conjunction with individual psychotherapy, they can be coded and billed directly to the patient. Just be sure the patients are informed that you will be doing this and get their written consent.

E/M codes will be used most frequently by those who care for patients in hospitals or partial hospital settings (99221–99239), provide inpatient consultations (99251–99263) (for Medicare, see p. 61), and/or provide patient services in nursing facilities (99301–99316). Home visits are covered by codes 99341–99350. See Chapter 4 for guidelines on the selection of E/M codes.

STEP 3: DOCUMENT YOUR SERVICES

The guidelines and recommendations for documenting services are covered in detail in Chapters 2–5. In Appendix F you will find vignettes illustrating the use of E/M codes, and in Appendix H you will find templates for documentation to support the selection of these codes.

STEP 4: SUBMIT THE CLAIM

You may recall the description of claims processing and the personnel involved from Chapter 7. The following suggestions will also help in the claims submission process:

- Claim forms must be filled out completely and legibly. **A legible signature is a vital part of this process.** Do not give the carrier a reason to return your claim; carriers take long enough to process clean claim forms. Time is money in the billing process.
- Send daily charges for each patient on separate forms. Although separate forms take slightly more time to complete, forms with multiple dates of service may cause confusion and are far more likely to be delayed in processing or returned.
- Consider electronic submission of claims if you are not already doing this. You will bypass both the carrier mailroom and claims examiners, thereby eliminating two sources of potential delay in the processing of your claims. Remember, however, that if you have been unaffected by HIPAA because you did not do any electronic transactions, if you file claims electronically, your practice will have to comply with HIPAA regulations (see Appendix B). This should not be a problem for most practices.
- If you submit a claim for an unusual service or use a code that has a modifier, include a brief explanatory note.

Insurance companies use sophisticated claims review software that includes clinical edits for CPT and ICD codes to process claims. Billing data flagged by these software edits are subject to special review, which often results in rejection of the claims or requests for additional information about the claims. At a minimum, payment is delayed.

Health information manager Andrea L. Albaum-Feinstein, M.D.A., R.R.A., developed a list of ways to avoid these edits. Doing the following checks, which are based on her list, before you send in claims may save you both time and money:

- Verify CPT and ICD codes and their descriptors. Claims review software makes it essential that clinicians be aware of annual coding updates. Because ICD-9-CM is now recognized as the universal diagnosis coding system for billing purposes (and its use is required under HIPAA), the few discrepancies between DSM-IV-TR and ICD-9-CM codes may on rare occasions cause problems in such software. Should this occur, American Psychiatric Association (APA) members should contact the APA's Managed Care Help Line at 800-343-4671 or hsf@psych.org for assistance. (It should be noted that in 2013 ICD-10 will become the officially mandated diagnosis code system, but DSM will continue to be compatible with ICD and psychiatrists will be able to continue using DSM for diagnoses.)
- Verify the clinical appropriateness of the ICD diagnosis code with the CPT procedure code (e.g., a psychiatric diagnosis is not compatible with a surgical procedure code).
- Verify the clinical appropriateness of the clinician's specialty (e.g., a psychiatrist is not expected to be performing surgery).
- Verify the clinical appropriateness of the patient's sex and age for the diagnosis and procedure (e.g., a male is not expected to have a diagnosis of pregnancy nor is a child to be given electroconvulsive therapy).
- If the CPT code for *unlisted service* is used, remember that an explanation for the use of this code and a description of the service should always accompany the claim.
- Verify which codes insurance companies (and Medicare and Medicaid) consider nonpayable. These codes vary according to the benefits policies of insurers. Examples might include CPT codes for telephone calls or cosmetic surgery.
- Verify the appropriateness of CPT category/subcategory service codes for both E/M and other services.
- Verify the appropriateness of the charge for a specific CPT code. Each insurance company has a range of values for payment based on the specific CPT procedural code. If the range for a service is between $75 and $100 and the clinician bills $200, the claim will be flagged.
- Verify that the CPT codes chosen do not conflict with coding instructions.
- Verify that you are not inappropriately bundling or unbundling CPT codes. *Bundling* is the practice of combining several procedures or services into one code when these services should be billed separately. *Unbundling* is the practice of billing for separate codes when one code for combined services should be used (i.e., charging for a psychotherapy session and for a separate medication management encounter on the same day when the correct code would be the appropriately timed psychotherapy code with E/M services).
- Select claims by various classifications—clinician, specialty, age, sex, or diagnostic or procedural codes—for internal quality assurance or utilization audits.

SUMMARY

As you code your claims, consider the following suggestions:

- Make coding a priority for the business component of your practice. The coding process affects your reimbursement, and proper coding prevents audits.

- Buy and use the CPT manual published annually by the American Medical Association.
- Keep in touch with your colleagues about coding and billing issues through the relevant committees of your professional association.
- Use codes appropriately; medical fraud is a very high priority of the U.S. Department of Justice.
- Code and bill for all services that you provide to patients regardless of local and/or national payer policies. The developing database of physician charges eventually may help practitioners change payment policies for more favorable reimbursement of mental health services.

QUESTIONS AND ANSWERS

Q. *Codes and documentation requirements keep changing. How can I keep up with the changes to be sure I am coding and documenting properly?*

A. Because the CPT Editorial Panel adds and modifies codes every year, you should obtain an updated version of the CPT manual each year. In addition, if you are a member of the APA, the CPT Coding Service and the Office of Healthcare Systems and Financing are available to assist you in answering specific coding questions (see Appendix L). Because documentation requirements follow the additions or modifications of codes, these same sources would be helpful to you in tracking the evolution of the documentation requirements.

Q. *I have continuous reimbursement problems with commercial payers/Medicare carriers/managed care organizations. What can I do?*

A. There are a number of steps you can take:

- Make sure all of your insurance forms are filled out accurately, completely, and legibly. If you have attachments to the insurance form, stamp or write on attachments "Please do not separate attachments."
- Contact your local professional society. It may be able to put you in touch with colleagues who have similar problems, assist you in assessing resources, sponsor legislation, and organize and sponsor legal actions.
- Ask your patients for assistance. Informing patients about your problems with their insurance companies is not unethical. Patients can help by talking to their employers' human resources departments and requesting reviews of their claims.
- APA members can call APA's Office of Healthcare Systems and Financing at 800-343-4671. Staff members have access to a wide range of resources to help you with third-party payers.

Q. *When I have questions about Medicare's reimbursement policies, whom should I call?*

A. Because Medicare is administered regionally by independent contractors, and because each contractor establishes some of its own reimbursement policies, you should contact your local Medicare contractor directly for information on reimbursement policies that affect your practice. APA members can call the Office of Healthcare Systems and Financing at 800-343-4671 if they need help finding out who their contractor is or solving problems that have arisen with that contractor.

9

FAQs and Problem Scenarios

Q. *When I see a patient specifically to discuss the use of medications for treatment, but the outcome is that I do not write a prescription because the patient has decided he or she does not want to take any drugs and we will reassess her need for them at a later date, is it still appropriate to use 90862?*

A. Yes, 90862 would still be the appropriate code, but you should be sure to note in your documentation how the decision was made not to prescribe anything. This should not be a frequent occurrence, especially for the same patient. If it happened on a regular basis, Medicare or another insurer might start to question the use of the medication management code and require documentation before a claim would be paid.

Q. *Can I use the appropriately timed psychotherapy code when I do a therapy session on the phone with a patient who is unable to come to the office?*

A. No. The psychotherapy codes specifically state that they are for face-to-face time with the patient. You might consider using code 90899, which is for "unlisted psychiatric service or procedure." Because this code is for an unlisted service, you will have to submit some kind of report with any claim that you file, explaining what the service was. Medicare will not cover therapy done over the telephone, and it would probably be wise to check with other insurers to see if they will cover it.

Q. *When I see a patient at an assisted living facility should I use inpatient or outpatient codes?*

A. Outpatient. For an assisted living facility you use a place of service code 13, which is for a residence. The inpatient place of service code is 21 and the office code is 11.

Q. *A patient is under the care of two nonphysician therapists, one for family therapy and another for individual therapy. After 2 weeks the patient is seen by a psychiatrist in the same practice to determine if medication is appropriate. A history is taken and a mental status examination is performed. The patient is* not placed on any medication, but the treatment plan states, "do not rule out possibility of medications in the future." Should this be coded as medication management (90862) or as an evaluation and management (E/M) code (99211–99213)?

A. Whether or not medication is prescribed, an E/M code would be the most appropriate code. The code chosen is based on the amount of work required. If the patient's case and current status are known to the psychiatrist, a 90862 might be appropriate, but if there has been a change in the patient's mental status and a psychiatric evaluation must be done, the appropriate E/M code should be selected.

Q. In a general medical teaching situation, the teaching physician must be present for the service to be billed to Medicare. However, for some psychiatry codes, the requirement of the teaching physician's presence can be met by observation through a one-way mirror or video equipment. Which codes does this not apply to?

A. According to Centers for Medicare and Medicaid Services guidelines, it does not apply to time-based codes, which would rule out the psychotherapy codes, both inpatient and outpatient.

Q. A psychiatrist admits a patient to inpatient services. The psychiatrist performs a psychiatric evaluation, reviews transfer records, writes medication orders, writes orders for level of observation required, orders laboratory work, and writes an initial treatment plan. The patient is later visited by a family practice physician who performs a physical examination and completes a document labeled "History and Physical Examination." This physician may write additional orders for medication and laboratory work. What are the appropriate codes for the two physicians to use?

A. The most appropriate codes for the psychiatrist to use would be 99221–99223, the initial hospital care E/M codes, the code to be chosen on the basis of the complexity of the case. Because the patient was apparently admitted for a psychiatric problem, use of the initial psychiatric evaluation code 90801 could also be appropriate. The family practitioner should use one of the appropriate inpatient E/M codes (99221–99223).

Q. If, on evaluation, it is determined that neither psychotherapy nor medication is needed, does this negate the use of 90801?

A. No, it does not.

Q. If a psychiatrist evaluates a patient and a trial of medication is indicated, but the patient's family physician does the prescribing, would it still be appropriate to use 90801?

A. Yes. However, a new patient office or other outpatient E/M code would be just as appropriate (99201–99205).

Q. A patient comes into the emergency department and the doctor there asks a psychiatrist to see the patient to assist with the evaluation and recommend outpatient psychiatric follow-up. The psychiatrist comes to the emergency de-

partment and documents the history of present illness, does a comprehensive history, performs a mental status examination, and provides the patient with contact numbers so he or she can arrange for therapy after leaving the hospital. What is the best way for the psychiatrist to code for this?

A. Either 90801 or one of the emergency department codes (99281–99285) is equally appropriate for this situation.

Q. *The attending psychiatrist of a psychiatric unit does a consult for a patient on the medical unit and uses code 99223. Several days later the patient is transferred to the psychiatric unit. May the psychiatrist who did the consult then bill a 99222 for initial hospital care, or must he or she use a follow-up code (e.g., 99232)?*

A. The psychiatrist should use an initial hospital care code for the first day in the psychiatric unit but would most likely use a lower level (99221 or 99222) because the patient database was already established during the consult.

Q. *In a teaching hospital, residents may spend as much as an hour with a psychiatric patient who has been in the hospital for several days, and then the supervising psychiatrist spends a lesser time with the patient, sometimes to discuss appropriate medications or comment on an intervention. Can the coding reflect the time that the resident spent with the patient?*

A. No, the resident's time is covered under Medicare Part A and is included in the hospital payment. The supervising psychiatrist may code only for the specific work he or she performs. The appropriate code to use is one of the subsequent inpatient codes (99231–99233). A 90862 may be used if the only service provided that same day was medication management.

Q. *A psychiatrist (Dr. B) met twice with the parents of a young man with substance abuse problems at the request of Dr. A, the psychiatrist their son was seeing at that time. Dr. B saw the parents twice and recommended an intervention for their son. The son was then transferred to the care of Dr. B. How should Dr. B code the visits with the parents?*

A. The appropriate code for the initial visit would be a 90801. The second visit should be coded as a second 90801 (a continuation of the initial evaluation) because it was required to complete the evaluation.

Q. *In hospital-based outpatient settings, the initial psychiatric interview evaluation, 90801, is often conducted in part by a registered nurse, physician's assistant, or social worker, with the psychiatrist then meeting with the patient face-to-face and confirming some of the history and examination. Then the psychiatrist and the other clinician collaborate on the documentation, which is reviewed and signed by the psychiatrist. Is there any issue with conducting and documenting for a 90801 in this manner?*

A. This is acceptable. However, it is important to keep in mind that the psychiatrist will be taking legal responsibility for the data supplied by the other clinician.

Q. *For discharge services, is it acceptable to document "discharge services more than 30 minutes" or "less than 30 minutes," because that is how the discharge day codes are defined in the CPT manual (hospital: 99238 and 99239; nursing facility 99315 and 99316)?*

A. No, you must document the actual time spent and code accordingly.

Q. *If a patient is transferred from intensive outpatient program (IOP) to a partial hospitalization program (PHP), and the psychiatrist admitting the patient to the PHP is different from the psychiatrist who admitted the patient to the IOP, is it appropriate for the PHP psychiatrist to bill a 90801?*

A. Yes.

Q. *A patient is admitted to a hospital by a psychiatrist who uses a 90801 for the initial evaluation. The patient returns several months later and is seen by a different psychiatrist. Is it appropriate for the second psychiatrist to also code 90801, even though only a few months have passed?*

A. Yes, because it is a new episode, and a new initial evaluation must be done.

Appendix A

The CPT Coding System

How It Came to Be, How It Changes

THE AMA CPT EDITORIAL PANEL

The responsibility for updating Current Procedural Terminology (CPT) rests with the American Medical Association (AMA) CPT Editorial Panel, which is composed of 15 physicians and 1 doctor of podiatric medicine. Ten physicians are nominated by the AMA, one of whom is appointed chair, and one member each is nominated by the American Hospital Association, the Blue Cross/Blue Shield Association, the Health Insurance Association of America, the AMA Healthcare Professionals Advisory Committee (HCPAC) (which is composed of nonphysician members of the CPT Advisory Committee), and the Centers for Medicare and Medicaid Services. In 1983, the AMA and the U.S. Department of Health and Human Services developed an agreement that stipulated that this panel of physicians has the sole authority to revise, update, or modify CPT. From 1991 until 2007 there was a psychiatrist on the CPT Editorial Panel, Tracy Gordy, M.D. He served as its chair for the last 9 of those years.

THE CPT ADVISORY COMMITTEE

The CPT Editorial Panel is supported in its work by the CPT Advisory Committee, whose members are practicing physicians nominated by the national medical specialty societies represented in the AMA's House of Delegates as well as representatives from other health provider associations. The CPT Advisory Committee now has more than 90 members, including representatives from the American Psychiatric Association (APA), the American Academy of Child and Adolescent Psychiatry, the American Psychological Association, the American Nurses Association, and the National Association of Social Workers. The primary purpose of the Advisory Committee is to serve as a technical resource for the CPT Editorial

Panel. The full committee meets annually, and work groups are formed as needed to address specific tasks on behalf of the panel. The committee's main role is to advise the panel on procedural coding and nomenclature relevant to each member's specialty. The committee also provides documentation on medical and surgical procedures and suggests revisions to CPT.

REQUESTS FOR UPDATING CPT

The process by which changes to the coding system are made is described by the AMA as "deliberate." A specific series of steps are followed when suggestions are received for revisions of CPT:

1. AMA staff physicians and coding experts evaluate all coding suggestions.
2. If the inquiry involves an issue that has been recently addressed by the CPT Editorial Panel, the requester is informed of the panel's interpretation.
3. If the request concerns a new issue, or if significant new information is received on an item that has been previously reviewed by the panel, the request is referred to the appropriate members of the CPT Advisory Committee. In most cases, CPT Advisory Committee members have a formal network of advisers from within their own subspecialties and generally serve as chairpersons of the subspecialty's coding, reimbursement, or medical service committee. (The APA's network of advisers comprises the APA's Committee on RBRVS, Codes, and Reimbursement, with the chairperson of the committee serving as the APA's representative to the CPT Advisory Committee.)
4. If the advisers who have been contacted agree that no new code or revision is needed, then AMA staff respond to the request with information on how existing codes should be used to report the procedure.
5. If the contacted advisers concur that a change should be made, or if two or more advisers disagree or give conflicting information, the issue is then referred to the CPT Editorial Panel for resolution. In making its decisions, the panel asks the following questions:

    a. Is this a service that a physician may perform or a hospital-provided service mandated to be reported to a payer?
    b. Has the procedure/service been generally accepted by the medical community as evidenced by:
        - Peer-reviewed medical literature?
        - Assessment of a nationally recognized technology assessment agency program?
        - Specialty society evaluation?
        - Other available information?
    c. Is this procedure/service in widespread use? If not, does it represent a significant advance in medical practice? If so, has it advanced beyond the research/investigative stage?
        - Data from medical literature and, as available, from third-party payers will be reviewed as applicable.

d. Is this procedure/service adequately described by an existing code?
  - Can an existing code be revised?
  - Can modifiers be used with an existing code?

e. Does the procedure/service represent a different method of performing a given procedure or service? Does the technique substantially alter the management or outcome of a problem or condition and warrant a separate code?

The CPT Editorial Panel meets quarterly and relies on evidence of procedural safety and effectiveness as presented by the requester and specialty society advisers in making its decisions. There is one very important caveat—inclusion of a procedure in CPT does not guarantee reimbursement.

The Medicare physician reimbursement system, the Resource-Based Relative Value Scale (RBRVS), has caused the addition of a step in the process of editing CPT. In collaboration with Centers for Medicare and Medicaid Services, the AMA has established a new committee—the RVS Update Committee (RUC)—whose purpose is to develop relative values for new or revised procedures. The RUC comprises physician representatives from 22 specialty societies in addition to a representative from the AMA, who serves as the chairperson and is a member of the CPT Editorial Panel. The RVS Update Committee was established in November 1991.

Appendix B

The Health Insurance Portability and Accountability Act (HIPAA)

INTRODUCTION

The Health Insurance Portability and Accountability Act of 1996 (HIPAA) was passed to address concerns arising from the increasing complexity of the medical delivery system and the increasing dependence of that system on electronic communications.

Many of these concerns had to do with the confidentiality of patients' personal information in the new electronic world. Although many states already had laws in place protecting patients' privacy, it was thought there should be a federal standard that would establish a minimum level of protection. In cases where state laws are more stringent than HIPAA in protecting patients' records and their access to them, those state laws take precedence over HIPAA. HIPAA mandates that the U.S. Department of Health and Human Services (DHHS) develop rules covering the transmission and confidentiality of individually identifiable health information, with which all entities covered under HIPAA must comply. The rule-making is ongoing.

The first two rules finalized under HIPAA were the Transactions Rule and the Privacy Rule. The Transactions Rule is intended to facilitate the ability to transfer health information accurately and efficiently, and the Privacy Rule was created to protect the confidentiality of patient information. The third rule that has been finalized is the Security Rule, which was created to protect the confidentiality of patient records kept on computers.

The underlying premise of the Privacy Rule is that a patient's individually identifiable health information belongs to the patient and that the patient has the right to gain access to that information and to control what is done with it.

Under the Transactions Rule, the DHHS created regulations that establish a uniform set of formats, code sets, and data requirements intended to permit the efficient, easily transferable, and secure electronic exchange of information for all healthcare administrative and financial transactions. The agency that administers the Medicare program, the Centers for Medicare and Medicaid Services (CMS), was charged with overseeing the implementation of the Transactions Rule. The Privacy Rule is administered by the DHHS Office for Civil Rights.

The Security Rule can be seen as an extension of the Privacy Rule: it requires that HIPAA-covered entities "protect against any reasonably anticipated threats or hazards to the security or integrity of protected health information, and protect against any reasonably anticipated uses and disclosures not permitted by the Privacy Rule and other more stringent laws."

Following the publication of the Transactions Rule (Standards for Electronic Transactions) and the Privacy Rule (Standards of Privacy for Individually Identifiable Health Information), both of which fall under the Administrative Simplification part of HIPAA, there was a great deal of concern about how compliance with these rules would affect the day-to-day practice of mental health clinicians.

In fact, compliance with HIPAA for mental health clinicians should not have proven to be all that difficult. Those providers who were seeing patients under the Medicare program were already using the code sets required by the Transactions Rule, and mental health clinicians were very likely to already have in place the confidentiality safeguards required by HIPAA because they have always been aware of the absolute necessity for maintaining the confidentiality of their patients' information.

THE TRANSACTIONS RULE

The Transactions Rule defines standards and establishes code sets and forms to be used for electronic transactions that involve the following kinds of healthcare information:

1. Claims or equivalent encounter information
2. Eligibility inquiries
3. Referral certification and authorization
4. Claims status inquiries
5. Enrollment and disenrollment information
6. Payment and remittance advice
7. Health plan premium payments
8. Coordination of benefits

The Transactions Rule code sets replaced the approximately 400 different formats that were in use for healthcare claims processing. These code sets simplify things for most providers. In the past, if they wanted to get paid, providers were forced to comply with whatever coding system the patient's insurer happened to be using. HIPAA also requires all insurers to use the same forms, which simplifies transactions with insurers as well.

The code sets required under the Transactions Rule are currently those that were already being used for filing claims with Medicare:

- **Procedure codes:** American Medical Association Current Procedural Terminology (CPT) and Healthcare Common Procedure Coding System codes
- **Diagnosis codes:** ICD-9-CM codes. *Note:* Clinicians should be able to continue to use DSM-IV-TR for diagnoses without experiencing difficulties, because almost all ICD-9-CM codes coincide with DSM-IV-TR codes.
- A new electronic data interchange standard, HIPAA 5010, will be required on January 1, 2012. By October 1, 2013, the diagnosis codes to be used under HIPAA 5010 will be from ICD-10-CM rather than the current ICD-9-CM.
- **Codes for drugs and biologicals:** National Drug Codes
- **Dental codes:** Code on Dental Procedures and Nomenclature for Dental Services

HIPAA also requires the use of uniform employer and provider identification numbers. Since May 23, 2008, all physicians and their corporations or the facilities where they work must be identified by a National Provider Identifier.

THE PRIVACY RULE

The Privacy Rule went into effect on April 14, 2003. It was enacted to address public concerns that the increased use of electronic technology and changes in the way healthcare is delivered could be undermining the confidentiality of the individually identifiable health information maintained and shared by clinicians, health insurance plans, and the other entities involved in patient care (however peripherally). The Privacy Rule established a federal floor of standards for the use and disclosure of patients' information. As previously mentioned, many states also have laws that deal with this issue, and in cases where the state law is more stringently protective of patients' rights, the state laws take precedence over the federal Privacy Rule. Contact your state medical society to find out whether the state laws in your jurisdiction preempt HIPAA.

Patients' Rights

Under the Privacy Rule your patients have statutory rights regarding their individually identifiable health information:

- You must give your patients written notice of their privacy rights and the privacy policies of your practice and how you will use, keep, and disclose their health information, and you must make a good-faith effort to obtain your patients' written acknowledgment that they have seen this notice.
- Patients must be able to get copies of their medical records and request amendments to those records within a stated time frame (usually 30 days). Patients do not have the right to see psychotherapy notes (see "Psychotherapy Notes" below).
- On patient request, you must provide your patients with a history of most disclosures of their medical records (there are some exceptions).
- You must obtain your patients' specific authorization for disclosures of their information other than for treatment, payment, and healthcare operations

(these three are considered to be "routine" uses). *Note:* Although HIPAA does not require that you obtain your patients' consent before disclosing their health information for treatment, payment, and healthcare operations, psychiatric ethics demand that you obtain written consent for these releases.

- Patients may request alternative means of communication of their protected information, for example, they may ask that you only contact them at a specific address or phone number.
- You generally cannot condition treatment of patients on obtaining their authorization for disclosure of their information for nonroutine uses.
- Your patients are authorized to complain about violations of the Privacy Rule to you, their health plan, or the Secretary of the DHHS.

Psychotherapy Notes

The writers of the Privacy Rule acknowledged that psychotherapy notes should be subject to a more stringent standard of confidentiality than other medical records. Psychotherapy notes are the only part of their files patients do not have access to. According to the rule, *psychotherapy notes* are specifically defined as the notes that are taken by a psychotherapist "documenting or analyzing the contents of a conversation during a private counseling session or a group, joint, or family counseling session and that are separate from the rest of the individual's medical record." Essentially, psychotherapy notes are the notations kept during therapy sessions that deal with the patient's personal life and the therapist's reactions, rather than with the patient's disorder. It is vital to understand that psychotherapy notes must be kept separate from the rest of the medical record (i.e., on a different sheet of paper) if they are to be protected as a separate entity. If psychotherapy notes cannot be separated from the rest of a patient's record, then they must be released with the rest of the record.

It is important to be clear about the definition of psychotherapy notes under HIPAA. Psychotherapy notes do *not* include references to medication prescribing and monitoring; session start and stop times; modality and frequency of treatment furnished; results of clinical tests; or any summary of the following items: diagnosis, symptoms, functional status, treatment plan, progress to date, and prognosis. All of this information is part of the medical record.

Minimum Necessary

The concept of minimum necessary disclosure is the rule for all routine disclosures of patients' individually identifiable information under HIPAA. However, when a patient gives authorization for a specific nonroutine disclosure, the concept of minimum necessary does not apply.

What a Clinician's Office Must Do to Be in Compliance With the Privacy Rule

To be in compliance with HIPAA, every practice must do the following:

- Have written privacy procedures that include administrative, physical, and technical safeguards establishing who has access to individually identifiable patient information, how this information is used within the practice, and when the information will and will not be disclosed to others.

- Ensure its business associates protect the privacy of health information, and train employees to comply with the Privacy Rule.
- Designate a person to serve as a privacy officer (a clinician in solo practice can be the privacy officer for the practice).
- Establish grievance procedures for patients who wish to inquire or complain about the privacy of their records.

THE SECURITY RULE

The Security Rule's requirements may be viewed as a standard for the protection of electronic health information that all providers, even those not covered by HIPAA, can be expected to meet or exceed. The Security Rule does not set forth any specific technology to be used to protect electronically maintained health information; rather, it demands that protections be in place against *reasonably anticipated* breaches of security. Most commercially available electronic health record systems should enable compliance with the HIPAA Security Rule.

Appendix C

Modifiers

Modifiers are two-digit numbers added to procedural codes (e.g., 90807–22) that indicate the procedure has been provided to the patient under special circumstances that do not alter the basic definition of the procedure. Without modifiers, many more procedural listings would be needed to represent a variety of circumstances. The complete list of modifiers can be found in Appendix A of the AMA CPT manual (CPT 2010 Professional Edition, pp. 529–533). The following are the modifiers most commonly used by psychiatrists and other mental health providers:

–22   Increased procedural services

This modifier is to be used when the work associated with the service provided is greater than that usually required for the listed procedure.

–25   Significant, separately identifiable evaluation and management service by the same physician on the same day of the procedure or other service

This modifier is used if the patient's condition changes on the day a service was provided and the condition requires a significant, separately identifiable evaluation and management service even though the diagnosis may be the same.

–26   Professional component

When procedures include a physician component and a technical component, the physician component can be reported separately by using this modifier.

–32   Mandated services

This modifier is used to report mandated consultations or services. An example of a mandated consultation is a second opinion for using electroconvulsive therapy. The confirmatory consultation codes **99271–99275** would be used with the addition of this modifier.

–52   Reduced services

This modifier is used to report a procedure that is reduced in work or time from that which is considered usual.

DOCUMENTATION REQUIREMENTS

When reporting modified procedures to insurance carriers, you must remember to explain to the carrier the special circumstances that necessitated the use of the modifier to improve your chances of being reimbursed. The explanation should be a short note describing, in a factual, jargon-free manner, 1) the patient's problem, 2) the treatment provided, 3) the time and effort, and 4) the medical necessity of the altered procedure. The following is an example of an explanatory note for the use of a modifier:

Extended Psychotherapy Session—**90807–22 (65 minutes)**

(Patient's name)
(ID number)
(Group number)
(Date of service)
(Your name and address)

Dear _____:

Mr. X was scheduled for a 50-minute psychotherapy session for the treatment of his depressive illness. Near the close of the session, he told me about the sudden onset of suicidal thoughts. These thoughts were of sufficient intensity to require an additional 15 minutes of work with Mr. X to review the symptoms and convince him of the necessity of hospitalization. The total time of the individual psychotherapy was 65 minutes.

Appendix D

Place of Service Codes for Medicare

Note: Some numbers are missing in what seems to be a consecutive list. That is because those numbers have not been assigned to any place of service (POS) as of 2010.

01 Pharmacy
03 School
04 Homeless shelter
05 Indian Health Service freestanding facility
06 Indian Health Service provider-based facility
07 Tribal 638 freestanding facility
08 Tribal 638 provider-based facility
11 Office
12 Home (private residence)
13 Assisted living facility
14 Group home
15 Mobile unit
16 Temporary lodging (any short-term accommodation—i.e., hotel, cruise ship, campground—that is not identified by any other POS code)
20 Urgent care facility
21 Inpatient hospital
22 Outpatient hospital
23 Emergency room—hospital
24 Ambulatory surgical center
25 Birthing center
26 Military treatment facility
31 Skilled nursing facility
32 Nursing facility
33 Custodial care facility

34   Hospice
41   Ambulance—land
42   Ambulance—land or water
49   Independent clinic
50   Federally qualified health center
51   Inpatient psychiatric facility
52   Psychiatric facility—partial hospitalization
53   Community mental health center
54   Intermediate care facility/mentally retarded
55   Residential substance abuse treatment facility
56   Psychiatric residential treatment center
57   Nonresidential substance abuse treatment facility
60   Mass immunization center
61   Comprehensive inpatient rehabilitation facility
62   Comprehensive outpatient rehabilitation facility
65   End-stage renal disease treatment facility
71   Public health clinic
72   Rural health clinic
81   Independent laboratory
99   Other place of service (not identified above)

Appendix E

1997 CMS Documentation Guidelines for Evaluation and Management Services (Abridged and Modified for Psychiatric Services)

I. INTRODUCTION

A. What Is Documentation and Why Is It Important?

Medical record documentation is required to record pertinent facts, findings, and observations about an individual's health history, including past and present illnesses, examinations, tests, treatments, and outcomes. The medical record chronologically documents the care of the patient and is an important element contributing to high-quality care. The medical record facilitates:

- the ability of the physician and other healthcare professionals to evaluate and plan the patient's immediate treatment, and to monitor his or her healthcare over time;
- communication and continuity of care among physicians and other healthcare professionals involved in the patient's care;
- accurate and timely claims review and payment;
- appropriate utilization review and quality of care evaluations; and
- collection of data that may be useful for research and education.

An appropriately documented medical record can reduce many of the "hassles" associated with claims processing and may serve as a legal document to verify the care provided, if necessary.

B. What Do Payers Want and Why?

Because payers have a contractual obligation to enrollees, they may require reasonable documentation that services are consistent with the insurance coverage provided. They may request information to validate:

- the site of service;
- the medical necessity and appropriateness of the diagnostic and/or therapeutic services provided; and/or
- that services provided have been accurately reported.

II. GENERAL PRINCIPLES OF MEDICAL RECORD DOCUMENTATION

The principles of documentation listed here are applicable to all types of medical and surgical services in all settings. For evaluation and management (E/M) services, the nature and amount of physician work and documentation varies by type of service, place of service, and the patient's status. The general principles listed here may be modified to account for these variable circumstances in providing E/M services.

1. The medical record should be complete and legible.
2. The documentation of each patient encounter should include:
   - reason for the encounter and relevant history, physical examination findings, and prior diagnostic test results;
   - assessment, clinical impression, or diagnosis;
   - plan for care; and
   - date and legible identity of the observer.
3. If not documented, the rationale for ordering diagnostic and other ancillary services should be easily inferred.
4. Past and present diagnoses should be accessible to the treating and/or consulting physician.
5. Appropriate health risk factors should be identified.
6. The patient's progress, response to and changes in treatment, and revision of diagnosis should be documented.
7. The Current Procedural Terminology (CPT) and ICD-9-CM codes reported on the health insurance claim form or billing statement should be supported by the documentation in the medical record.

III. DOCUMENTATION OF E/M SERVICES

This publication provides definitions and documentation guidelines for the three key components of E/M services and for visits that consist predominantly of counseling or coordination of care. The three *key* components—history, examination, and medical decision making—appear in the descriptors for office and other outpatient services, hospital observation services, hospital inpatient services, consultations, emergency department services, nursing facility services, domiciliary care services, and home services. While some of the text of CPT has been repeated in this publication, the reader should refer to CPT for the complete descriptors for E/M services and instructions for selecting a level of service. Documentation guidelines are identified by the symbol • *DG.*

The descriptors for the levels of E/M services recognize seven components that are used in defining the levels of E/M services:

- History
- Examination
- Medical decision making
- Counseling
- Coordination of care
- Nature of presenting problem
- Time

The first three of these components (i.e., history, examination, and medical decision making) are the key components in selecting the level of E/M services. In the case of visits that consist predominantly of counseling or coordination of care, time is the key or controlling factor to qualify for a particular level of E/M service.

Because the level of E/M service is dependent on two or three key components, performance and documentation of one component (e.g., examination) at the highest level does not necessarily mean that the encounter in its entirety qualifies for the highest level of E/M service.

These Documentation Guidelines for E/M services reflect the needs of the typical adult population. For certain groups of patients, the recorded information may vary slightly from that described here. Specifically, the medical records of infants, children, adolescents, and pregnant women may have additional or modified information recorded in each history and examination area.

As an example, newborn records may include under history of the present illness the details of mother's pregnancy and the infant's status at birth; social history will focus on family structure; and family history will focus on congenital anomalies and hereditary disorders in the family. In addition, the content of a pediatric examination will vary with the age and development of the child. Although not specifically defined in these documentation guidelines, these patient group variations on history and examination are appropriate.

A. Documentation of History

The levels of E/M services are based on four types of history (problem focused, expanded problem focused, detailed, and comprehensive). Each type of history includes some or all of the following elements:

- Chief complaint (CC)
- History of present illness (HPI)
- Review of systems (ROS)
- Past, family, and/or social history (PFSH)

The extent of HPI, ROS, and PFSH that is obtained and documented is dependent on clinical judgment and the nature of the presenting problem(s).

The chart below shows the progression of the elements required for each type of history. To qualify for a given type of history all three elements in the table must be met. (A CC is indicated at all levels.)

History of present illness (HPI)	Review of systems (ROS)	Past, family, and/or social history (PFSH)	Type of history
Brief	N/A	N/A	Problem focused
Brief	Problem pertinent	N/A	Expanded problem focused
Extended	Extended	Pertinent	Detailed
Extended	Complete	Complete	Comprehensive

- *DG: The CC, ROS, and PFSH may be listed as separate elements of history or may be included in the description of the history of the present illness.*

- *DG: An ROS and/or a PFSH obtained during an earlier encounter does not need to be re-recorded if there is evidence that the physician reviewed and updated the previous information. This may occur when a physician updates his or her own record or in an institutional setting or group practice where many physicians use a common record. The review and update may be documented by*

    - *describing any new ROS and/or PFSH information or noting there has been no change in the information; and*
    - *noting the date and location of the earlier ROS and/or PFSH.*

- *DG: The ROS and/or PFSH may be recorded by ancillary staff or on a form completed by the patient. To document that the physician reviewed the information, there must be a notation supplementing or confirming the information recorded by others.*

- *DG: If the physician is unable to obtain a history from the patient or other source, the record should describe the patient's condition or other circumstance that precludes obtaining a history.*

Definitions and specific documentation guidelines for each of the elements of history are listed in the following sections.

CHIEF COMPLAINT (CC)

The CC is a concise statement describing the symptom, problem, condition, diagnosis, physician recommended return, or other factor that is the reason for the encounter, usually stated in the patient's words.

- *DG: The medical record should clearly reflect the CC.*

HISTORY OF PRESENT ILLNESS (HPI)

The HPI is a chronological description of the development of the patient's present illness from the first sign and/or symptom or from the previous encounter to the present. It includes the following elements:

- Location
- Quality
- Severity
- Duration
- Timing
- Context
- Modifying factors
- Associated signs and symptoms

Brief and *extended* HPIs are distinguished by the amount of detail needed to accurately characterize the clinical problem(s).

A *brief* HPI consists of one to three elements of the HPI.

- *DG: The medical record should describe one to three elements of the present illness.*

An *extended* HPI consists of at least four elements of the HPI or the status of at least three chronic or inactive conditions.

- *DG: The medical record should describe at least four elements of the present illness or the status of at least three chronic or inactive conditions.*

REVIEW OF SYSTEMS (ROS)

An ROS is an inventory of body systems obtained through a series of questions seeking to identify signs and/or symptoms that the patient may be experiencing or has experienced.

For purposes of the ROS, the following systems are recognized:

- Constitutional symptoms (e.g., fever, weight loss)
- Eyes
- Ears, nose, mouth, throat
- Cardiovascular
- Respiratory
- Gastrointestinal
- Genitourinary
- Musculoskeletal
- Integumentary (skin and/or breast)
- Neurological
- Psychiatric
- Endocrine
- Hematological/Lymphatic
- Allergic/Immunologic

A *problem pertinent* ROS inquires about the system directly related to the problem(s) identified in the HPI.

- *DG: The patient's positive responses and pertinent negatives for the system related to the problem should be documented.*

An *extended* ROS inquires about the system directly related to the problem(s) identified in the HPI and a limited number of additional systems.

- *DG: The patient's positive responses and pertinent negatives for two to nine systems should be documented.*

A *complete* ROS inquires about the system(s) directly related to the problem(s) identified in the HPI *plus* all additional body systems.

- *DG: At least 10 organ systems must be reviewed. Those systems with positive or pertinent negative responses must be individually documented. For the remaining systems, a notation indicating all other systems are negative is permissible. In the absence of such a notation, at least 10 systems must be individually documented.*

PAST, FAMILY, AND/OR SOCIAL HISTORY (PFSH)

The PFSH consists of a review of three areas:

- Past history (the patient's past experiences with illnesses, operations, injuries, and treatments)
- Family history (a review of medical events in the patient's family, including diseases that may be hereditary or place the patient at risk)
- Social history (an age-appropriate review of past and current activities)

For certain categories of E/M services that include only an interval history, it is not necessary to record information about the PFSH. Those categories are subsequent hospital care, follow-up inpatient consultations, and subsequent nursing facility care.

A *pertinent* PFSH is a review of the history area(s) directly related to the problem(s) identified in the HPI.

- *DG: At least one specific item from any of the three history areas must be documented for a pertinent PFSH.*

A *complete* PFSH is of a review of two or all three of the PFSH history areas, depending on the category of the E/M service. A review of all three history areas is required for services that by their nature include a comprehensive assessment or reassessment of the patient. A review of two of the three history areas is sufficient for other services.

- *DG: At least one specific item from two of the three history areas must be documented for a complete PFSH for the following categories of E/M services: office or other outpatient services, established patient; emergency department; domiciliary care, established patient; and home care, established patient.*

♦ *DG: At least one specific item from each of the three history areas must be documented for a complete PFSH for the following categories of E/M services: office or other outpatient services, new patient; hospital observation services; hospital inpatient services, initial care; consultations; comprehensive nursing facility assessments; domiciliary care, new patient; and home care, new patient.*

B. Documentation of Examination

The levels of E/M services are based on four types of examination:

- *Problem focused*—A limited examination of the affected body area or organ system.
- *Expanded problem focused*—A limited examination of the affected body area or organ system and any other symptomatic or related body area(s) or organ system(s).
- *Detailed*—An extended examination of the affected body area(s) or organ system(s) and any other symptomatic or related body area(s) or organ system(s).
- *Comprehensive*—A general multisystem examination or complete examination of a single organ system and other symptomatic or related body area(s) or organ system(s).

These types of examinations have been defined for general multisystem and the following single organ systems:

- Cardiovascular
- Ears, nose, mouth, and throat
- Eyes
- Genitourinary (female)
- Genitourinary (male)
- Hematological/Lymphatic/Immunological
- Musculoskeletal
- Neurological
- **Psychiatric**
- Respiratory
- Skin

A general multisystem examination or a single organ system examination may be performed by any physician regardless of specialty. The type (general multisystem or single organ system) and content of examination are selected by the examining physician and are based upon clinical judgment, the patient's history, and the nature of the presenting problem(s).

The content and documentation requirements for each type and level of examination are summarized here and described in detail in the tables that appear later in this appendix. In the first table (see pp. 123), organ systems and body areas recognized by CPT for purposes of describing examinations are shown in the left column. The content, or individual elements, of the examination pertaining to that body area or organ system are identified by bullets (•) in the right column.

Parenthetical examples "(e.g., ...)" have been used for clarification and to provide guidance regarding documentation. Documentation for each element must satisfy any numeric requirements (such as "Measurement of *any three of the following seven...*") included in the description of the element. Elements with multiple components but with no specific numeric requirement (such as "Examination of *liver* and *spleen*") require documentation of at least one component. It is possible for a given examination to be expanded beyond what is defined here. When that occurs, findings related to the additional systems and/or areas should be documented.

- *DG: Specific abnormal and relevant negative findings of the examination of the affected or symptomatic body area(s) or organ system(s) should be documented. A notation of "abnormal" without elaboration is insufficient.*

- *DG: Abnormal or unexpected findings of the examination of any asymptomatic body area(s) or organ system(s) should be described.*

- *DG: A brief statement or notation indicating "negative" or "normal" is sufficient to document normal findings related to unaffected area(s) or asymptomatic organ system(s).*

[Deleted: Guidelines for "General Multi-System Examinations"]

Single Organ System Examinations

The single organ system examinations recognized by CPT are described in detail. [*Authors' note:* We are only including the psychiatric examination.] Variations among these examinations in the organ systems and body areas identified in the left columns and in the elements of the examinations described in the right columns reflect differing emphases among specialties. To qualify for a given level of single organ system examination, the following content and documentation requirements should be met:

- *Problem focused examination*—Should include performance and documentation of one to five elements identified by a bullet (•), whether in a box with a shaded or unshaded border.
- *Expanded problem focused examination*—Should include performance and documentation of at least six elements identified by a bullet (•), whether in a box with a shaded or unshaded border.
- *Detailed examination*—Examinations other than the eye and psychiatric examinations should include performance and documentation of at least 12 elements identified by a bullet (•), whether in box with a shaded or unshaded border.

   Eye and psychiatric examinations should include the performance and documentation of at least nine elements identified by a bullet (•), whether in a box with a shaded or unshaded border.

- *Comprehensive examination*—Should include performance of all elements identified by a bullet (•), whether in a shaded or unshaded box. Documentation of every element in each box with a shaded border and at least one element in each box with an unshaded border is expected.

CONTENT AND DOCUMENTATION REQUIREMENTS
[DELETED: CONTENT AND DOCUMENTATION REQUIREMENTS FOR GENERAL MULTI-SYSTEM EXAMINATION AND ALL SINGLE-SYSTEM REQUIREMENTS OTHER THAN PSYCHIATRY]

PSYCHIATRIC EXAMINATION

SYSTEM/ BODY AREA	ELEMENTS OF EXAMINATION
Constitutional	• Measurement of any **three of the following seven** vital signs: 1) sitting or standing blood pressure, 2) supine blood pressure, 3) pulse rate and regularity, 4) respiration, 5) temperature, 6) height, 7) weight (may be measured and recorded by ancillary staff) • General appearance of patient (e.g., development, nutrition, body habitus, deformities, attention to grooming)
Head and Face	
Eyes	
Ears, Nose, Mouth, and Throat	
Neck	
Respiratory	
Cardiovascular	
Chest (Breasts)	
Gastrointestinal (Abdomen)	
Genitourinary	
Lymphatic	
Musculoskeletal	• Assessment of muscle strength and tone (e.g., flaccid, cog wheel, spastic) with notation of any atrophy and abnormal movements • Examination of gait and station
Extremities	
Skin	
Neurological	

PSYCHIATRIC EXAMINATION *(CONTINUED)*	
SYSTEM/ BODY AREA	**ELEMENTS OF EXAMINATION**
Psychiatric	• Description of speech, including rate, volume, articulation, coherence, and spontaneity with notation of abnormalities (e.g., perseveration, paucity of language) • Description of thought processes, including rate of thoughts; content of thoughts (e.g., logical vs. illogical, tangential); abstract reasoning; and computation • Description of associations (e.g., loose, tangential, circumstantial, intact) • Description of abnormal or psychotic thoughts, including hallucinations, delusions, preoccupation with violence, homicidal or suicidal ideation, and obsessions • Description of the patient's judgment (e.g., concerning everyday activities and social situations) and insight (e.g., concerning psychiatric condition) Complete mental status examination, including • Orientation to time, place, and person • Recent and remote memory • Attention span and concentration • Language (e.g., naming objects, repeating phrases) • Fund of knowledge (e.g., awareness of current events, past history, vocabulary) • Mood and affect (e.g., depression, anxiety, agitation, hypomania, lability)

CONTENT AND DOCUMENTATION REQUIREMENTS	
LEVEL OF EXAMINATION	**PERFORM AND DOCUMENT**
Problem focused	**One to five** elements identified by a bullet.
Expanded problem focused	**At least six** elements identified by a bullet.
Detailed	**At least nine** elements identified by a bullet.
Comprehensive	Perform **all** elements identified by a bullet; document every element in each box with a shaded border and at least one element in each box with an unshaded border.

C. Documentation of the Complexity of Medical Decision Making

The levels of E/M services recognize four types of medical decision making: straightforward, low complexity, moderate complexity, and high complexity. *Medical decision making* refers to the complexity of establishing a diagnosis and/ or selecting a management option as measured by:

- the number of possible diagnoses and/or the number of management options that must be considered;
- the amount and/or complexity of medical records, diagnostic tests, and/or other information that must be obtained, reviewed, and analyzed; and
- the risk of significant complications, morbidity, and/or mortality, as well as comorbidities, associated with the patient's presenting problem(s), the diagnostic procedure(s) and/or the possible management options.

The following chart shows the progression of the elements required for each level of medical decision making. To qualify for a given type of decision making, **two of the three elements in the table must be either met or exceeded.**

Number of diagnoses or management options	Amount or complexity of data to be reviewed	Risk of complications and/or morbidity or mortality	Type of decision making
Minimal	Minimal or none	Minimal	*Straightforward*
Limited	Limited	Low	*Low complexity*
Multiple	Moderate	Moderate	*Moderate complexity*
Extensive	Extensive	High	*High complexity*

Each of the elements of medical decision making is described below.

Number of Diagnoses or Management Options

The number of possible diagnoses and/or the number of management options that must be considered is based on the number and types of problems addressed during the encounter, the complexity of establishing a diagnosis, and the management decisions that are made by the physician.

Generally, decision making with respect to a diagnosed problem is easier than that for an identified but undiagnosed problem. The number and type of diagnostic tests employed may be an indicator of the number of possible diagnoses. Problems that are improving or resolving are less complex than those that are worsening or failing to change as expected. The need to seek advice from others is another indicator of the complexity of diagnostic or management problems.

- *DG: For each encounter, an assessment, clinical impression, or diagnosis should be documented. It may be explicitly stated or implied in documented decisions regarding management plans and/or further evaluation.*

  - *For a presenting problem with an established diagnosis, the record should reflect whether the problem is a) improved, well controlled, resolving, or resolved or b) inadequately controlled, worsening, or failing to change as expected.*

  - *For a presenting problem without an established diagnosis, the assessment or clinical impression may be stated in the form of differential diagnoses or as a "possible," "probable," or "rule out" (R/O) diagnosis.*

- *DG: The initiation of, or changes in, treatment should be documented. Treatment includes a wide range of management options including patient instructions, nursing instructions, therapies, and medications.*

- *DG: If referrals are made, consultations requested, or advice sought, the record should indicate to whom or where the referral or consultation is made or from whom the advice is requested.*

AMOUNT AND COMPLEXITY OF DATA TO BE REVIEWED

The amount and complexity of data to be reviewed are based on the types of diagnostic testing ordered or reviewed. A decision to obtain and review old medical records and/or obtain history from sources other than the patient increases the amount and complexity of data to be reviewed.

Discussion of contradictory or unexpected test results with the physician who performed or interpreted the test is an indication of the complexity of data being reviewed. On occasion the physician who ordered a test may personally review the image, tracing, or specimen to supplement information from the physician who prepared the test report or interpretation; this is another indication of the complexity of data being reviewed.

- *DG: If a diagnostic service (test or procedure) is ordered, planned, scheduled, or performed at the time of the E/M encounter, the type of service (e.g., laboratory work or X-ray) should be documented.*

- *DG: The review of laboratory, radiology, and/or other diagnostic tests should be documented. A simple notation such as "white blood cells elevated" or "chest X-ray unremarkable" is acceptable. Alternatively, the review may be documented by initialing and dating the report containing the test results.*

- *DG: A decision to obtain old records or to obtain additional history from the family, caretaker, or other source to supplement that obtained from the patient should be documented.*

- *DG: Relevant findings from the review of old records and/or the receipt of additional history from the family, caretaker, or other source to supplement that obtained from the patient should be documented. If there is no relevant information beyond that already obtained, that fact should be documented. A notation of "old records reviewed" or "additional history obtained from family" without elaboration is insufficient.*

- *DG: The results of discussion of laboratory, radiology, or other diagnostic tests with the physician who performed or interpreted the study should be documented.*

- *DG: The direct visualization and independent interpretation of an image, tracing, or specimen previously or subsequently interpreted by another physician should be documented.*

RISK OF SIGNIFICANT COMPLICATIONS, MORBIDITY, AND/OR MORTALITY

The risk of significant complications, morbidity, and/or mortality is based on the risks associated with the presenting problem(s), the diagnostic procedure(s), and the possible management options.

- *DG: Comorbidities/Underlying diseases or other factors that increase the complexity of medical decision making by increasing the risk of complications, morbidity, and/or mortality should be documented.*

- *DG: If a surgical or invasive diagnostic procedure is ordered, planned, or scheduled at the time of the E/M encounter, the type of procedure (e.g., laparoscopy) should be documented.*

- *DG: If a surgical or invasive diagnostic procedure is performed at the time of the E/M encounter, the specific procedure should be documented.*

- *DG: The referral for or decision to perform a surgical or invasive diagnostic procedure on an urgent basis should be documented or implied.*

The table on p. 128 may be used to help determine whether the risk of significant complications, morbidity, and/or mortality is *minimal, low, moderate,* or *high*. Because the determination of risk is complex and not readily quantifiable, the table includes common clinical examples rather than absolute measures of risk. The assessment of risk of the presenting problem(s) is based on the risk related to the disease process anticipated between the present encounter and the next one. The assessment of risk of selecting diagnostic procedures and management options is based on the risk during and immediately following any procedures or treatment. **The highest level of risk in any one category (presenting problem[s], diagnostic procedure[s], or management options) determines the overall risk.**

D. Documentation of an Encounter Dominated by Counseling or Coordination of Care

In the case in which counseling and/or coordination of care dominates (more than 50%) the physician/patient and/or family encounter (face-to-face time in the office or other or outpatient setting, floor/unit time in the hospital or nursing facility), time is considered the key or controlling factor to qualify for a particular level of E/M services.

- *DG: If the physician elects to report the level of service based on counseling and/ or coordination of care, the total length of time of the encounter (face-to-face or floor time, as appropriate) should be documented, and the record should describe the counseling and/or activities to coordinate care.*

TABLE OF RISK
(MODIFIED FOR PSYCHIATRY FROM THE 1997 CMS GUIDELINES)

LEVEL OF RISK	PRESENTING PROBLEM(S)	DIAGNOSTIC PROCEDURE(S) ORDERED	MANAGEMENT OPTIONS SELECTED
Minimal	1 self-limited problem (e.g., medication side effect)	Laboratory tests requiring venipuncture Urinalysis	Reassurance
Low	2 or more self-limited or minor problems; or 1 stable chronic illness (e.g., well-controlled depressions); or Acute uncomplicated illness (e.g., exacerbation of anxiety disorder)	Psychological testing Skull film	Psychotherapy Environmental intervention (e.g., agency, school, vocational placement) Referral for consultation (e.g., physician, social worker)
Moderate	1 or more chronic illnesses with mild exacerbation, progression, or side effects of treatment; or 2 or more stable chronic illnesses; or Undiagnosed new problem with uncertain prognosis (e.g., psychosis)	Electroencephalogram Neuropsychological testing	Prescription drug management Open-door seclusion ECT, inpatient, outpatient, routine; no comorbid medical conditions
High	1 or more chronic illnesses with severe exacerbation, progression, or side effect of treatment (e.g., schizophrenia); or Acute illness with threat to life (e.g., suicidal or homicidal ideation)	Lumbar puncture Suicide risk assessment	Drug therapy requiring intensive monitoring (e.g., tapering diazepam for patient in withdrawal) Closed-door seclusion Suicide observation ECT; patient has comorbid medical condition (e.g., cardiovascular disease) Rapid intramuscular neuroleptic administration Pharmacological restraint (e.g., droperidol)

Vignettes for Evaluation and Management Codes

OFFICE VISIT, NEW PATIENT

99203   A 27-year-old woman with a history of depression who is visiting the area is seen in an initial office visit. She is currently under treatment in her hometown. History taking focuses on a review of her past psychiatric history, present illness, and interval history since her last visit to her treating psychiatrist. Her medication history is reviewed, as is her side-effect history. A mental status examination focuses on her current affective state, ability to attend and concentrate, and insight. A prescription for an antidepressant is provided, along with education on its use and side effects.

       Explanation for code choice: Although a new patient to the examining psychiatrist, this patient has an existing treatment source. The psychiatrist obtains a detailed history and performs a detailed mental status examination. (A detailed history requires a detailed [two to nine elements] review of symptoms.) The provision of a prescription requires medical decision making of low complexity.

99205   A 38-year-old man brought by his parents for evaluation of paranoid delusions and alcohol abuse is seen in an initial office visit. History taking focuses on the family history of mental illness. The past medical and psychiatric history, history of present illness, and social history of the patient are taken. The results of a mental status examination reveal a poorly groomed individual, poor eye contact, no spontaneity to speech, flat affect, no hallucinations, paranoid delusions about the police, no suicidal/homicidal ideation, and intact cognitive status. The patient has no history of current medical problems. The patient denies alcohol use. The parents are interviewed and provide a history of the patient that includes at least 5 years of binge drinking. Routine blood studies are ordered. The patient's vital signs are taken. A prescription for a neuroleptic is given, and education about medication is provided to the patient and the parents. Referrals to a dual-diagnosis treatment program and Alcoholics Anonymous are made.

Explanation for code choice: This initial evaluation requires complex medical decision making because of the psychotic symptoms in the context of alcohol abuse. The psychiatrist must complete a comprehensive history and examination. The comprehensive history includes a complete review of systems.

OFFICE VISIT, ESTABLISHED PATIENT

99213   A 42-year-old male established patient with a history of bipolar II disorder, last seen 2 months prior, is seen for an office visit. Interval history taking focuses on the presence/absence of symptoms, the patient's level of social/vocational function, and the patient's adherence to the medication regimen. A mental status examination focuses on the patient's affective state. The patient's lithium blood level is reviewed. The side effects of the medication are reviewed, and prescriptions for the same medications are provided.

Explanation for code choice: In order to make a decision about medications, the psychiatrist must do an expanded problem-focused history and examination. An expanded problem-focused history includes one to three elements of a review of systems. The actual medical decision to continue the medication regimen is of low complexity.

HOSPITAL INPATIENT SERVICES—INITIAL HOSPITAL CARE

99221   A 32-year-old woman is seen for initial hospital care. The woman had been discharged from the same psychiatric unit 3 days earlier after a 5-day stay precipitated by threats of suicide in the context of alcohol intoxication. The patient had received diagnoses of adjustment disorder with depressed mood and suicidal ideation, alcohol abuse, and mixed personality disorder with borderline features. Her interval history revealed that the patient had returned home after discharge from the hospital and within 24 hours became involved in verbally violent arguments with her husband, drank an unspecified amount of vodka, and threatened to kill him. Her blood alcohol level in the emergency department is 160 mg/dL. The results of a physical examination are within normal limits, as are the results of the remainder of the laboratory studies. The results of a toxicology screening are negative. The mental status examination reveals a patient who is crying, angry, and accusing her husband of infidelity. She is difficult to redirect, and her affect is labile and irritable. Her mood is depressed. She shows no psychotic symptoms and is cognitively intact. She demonstrates little to no insight. The patient is admitted to the hospital voluntarily. The social work staff is asked to provide an evaluation of the husband and the family situation. Discharge planning is begun.

Explanation for code choice: The lowest level of initial hospital care is appropriate because this is a readmission with no change in the history database and because the medical decision making is straightforward.

99222   A 40-year-old man discharged 12 days before the current admission with a diagnosis of schizophrenia had been given instructions to attend follow-up visits at an outpatient clinic to monitor his neuroleptic medication. He now presents with auditory hallucinations and paranoid ideation with violent thoughts toward his neighbors. His interval history reveals that he never attended the outpatient clinic and that he immediately discontinued taking the neuroleptic medication after discharge. The patient's brother reports that the patient's symptoms reappeared 4 days before the current admission. The patient also has a history of diabetes mellitus controlled by oral medications and had discontinued taking his diabetes medication. A mental status examination reveals a poorly groomed individual with auditory hallucinations that are threatening toward the patient and paranoid delusions that involve neighbors trying to hurt him. He admits to violent thoughts toward his neighbors and states that he might have to harm or kill them. He appears to be cognitively intact. A physical examination reveals a moderately obese individual. The results of his laboratory studies are normal except for an elevated glucose level. The results of repeat finger-stick tests indicate glucose levels above 400 mg/dL. A new neuroleptic regimen is begun for the patient. The treatment team devises a strategy to help the patient's family assist him in adhering to this regimen after discharge.

Explanation for code choice: Although this case is also a readmission, the nature of the presenting problem involves psychotic symptoms, violent thoughts, and symptomatic diabetes. The level of history taking and examination are comprehensive, and the medical decision making is moderately complex.

99223   Initial psychiatric hospital services are provided for a 17-year-old female transferred from the medical intensive care unit after treatment for ingestion of a large amount of acetaminophen and aspirin. Her family history reveals that her mother and a maternal uncle have been treated for depression. The patient has been doing poorly in school for 6 months and has been experimenting with drugs and alcohol. She has been rebellious at home, and 2 months ago she reported that she might be pregnant. One week before her admission, her boyfriend of 1 year left her for another schoolmate. She has no history of significant medical or surgical problems. Her last menstrual period was 3 weeks ago. The patient is admitted voluntarily. A mental status examination reveals a barely cooperative, sullen teenager whose speech is not spontaneous but is logical and coherent. She shows no psychotic symptoms. The patient refuses to comment on current suicidal thoughts or ideation. She is cognitively intact. The results of a physical examination and laboratory tests are all within normal limits. The social work staff is asked to assess the patient's family situation. The patient is placed on close observation as a suicide precaution.

Explanation for code choice: Suicidal behaviors always require highly complex medical decision making supported by a comprehensive history and comprehensive mental status examination. Be sure to complete a full review of systems.

99223   Initial hospital care is provided for a 35-year-old woman with a 3-month history of withdrawn, bizarre behavior. Two days before her admission she became disorganized and aggressive toward her family and started talking to herself. Her family history reveals a maternal grandfather with a diagnosis of schizophrenia. The patient had two prior episodes of psychosis and had received a diagnosis of schizophrenia. She dropped out of treatment 5–6 months ago, and since then she has not taken any medications. There are no current medical or surgical problems. The patient is admitted involuntarily. The results of a mental status examination reveal the patient to be uncooperative and poorly groomed and to make poor eye contact. Her speech is rambling and tangential. The patient appears to be responding to internal stimuli and is easily distracted and blocked. Her affect is flat and blunted. The patient is oriented to time, place, and person. The results of a physical examination and laboratory tests are within normal limits. The patient is placed on every-15-minute observation status. She is assessed for neuroleptic treatment. The social work staff is asked to assess the family situation. The occupational therapy/recreational therapy staff is asked to assess the patient's ability to perform activities of daily living.

Explanation for code choice: This is an example of a typical admission for a patient with a major psychiatric disorder and severe acute symptoms. The history and mental status examination must be comprehensive. A complete review of systems is required, and the medical decision making is highly complex.

99223   Initial hospital care is provided for an 8-year-old boy whose parents requested admission because of a 1-week history of repeated attempts to cut and hit himself. The patient's family history reveals that his father is in treatment for bipolar disorder. The patient is the second of three children. The siblings are reported to be doing well. The parents admit to having recent marital problems for which they have sought counseling. The patient is described as generally well behaved but moody with a bad temper. His schoolwork has been deteriorating for the past 3 months, and there have been reports of minor behavioral misconduct. One week before admission, the parents denied the patient a puppy. Since then he has been out of control and has been cutting, scratching, and hitting himself. A mental status examination reveals a withdrawn, depressed-appearing child who answers all questions with yes or no. He is cognitively intact. A physical examination reveals scratches and bruises over the patient's arms and legs. The results of laboratory studies are within normal limits. The social work staff is asked to begin a family assessment. The patient is placed on close observation.

Explanation for code choice: The out-of-control self-harm behavior requires highly complex medical decision making supported by a complete review of systems and a comprehensive history and examination.

99223   Initial hospital care is provided for a 75-year-old man with a 2-month history of depression, a 2-week history of auditory hallucinations, and recent suicidal ideation. The patient has a history of diabetes mellitus and is dehydrated. The psychiatric history focuses on past history of episodes of depression, family history of depression, and the patient's current social support system. A mental status examination reveals poor grooming, poor eye contact, lack of spontaneity, slowed speech, psychomotor retardation, depressed affect, present suicidal ideation with no plan, and auditory hallucinations telling the patient that he is no good. The patient is cognitively intact. The patient is admitted voluntarily. A medical consultation is requested. Complete blood count, SMA-12, and thyroid laboratory tests are ordered. The patient and the family are instructed about the probable need for electroconvulsive therapy. The consent process for electroconvulsive therapy is explained, and signatures are obtained. Exploration of discharge placement is begun. The patient is placed on close observation as a suicide precaution.

Explanation for code choice: Severe depression with psychotic symptoms and suicidal ideation in an elderly patient requires a comprehensive history and examination as well as a complete review of systems. Treatment considerations, taking into account medical comorbidities and including electroconvulsive therapy, demand highly complex medical decision making.

HOSPITAL INPATIENT SERVICES— SUBSEQUENT HOSPITAL CARE

99231   A 14-year-old female admitted for depression and suicidal ideation is seen in a subsequent hospital visit. The patient has been in the hospital for 12 days and is behaviorally stable. Her condition is improving. The attending psychiatrist interviews the patient; meets with the treatment team; reviews notes prepared by nursing, occupational therapy/recreational therapy, and social work staff; writes an order for as-needed medication for headache; and writes the daily progress note.

Explanation for code choice: This level of subsequent hospital care is appropriate because the patient is stable and approaching discharge. The medical decision making for this day's work is straightforward.

99232   A 36-year-old man admitted for hallucinations and delusions and now in his third hospital day is seen for a subsequent hospital visit. The attending psychiatrist interviews the patient, takes an interval history, does a mental status examination, and then meets with the treatment team. The team reviews notes prepared by nursing, occupational therapy/recreational therapy, and social work staff. The attending psychiatrist orders an increase in the patient's neuroleptic medication. The attending psychiatrist discusses discharge planning with social work staff, talks with the patient's mother by phone, and writes the daily progress note.

Explanation for code choice: This example of subsequent hospital care is typical of a mid-hospital-course day of work. The history and examination are at the expanded problem-focused level, and the medical decision making is moderately complex. The expanded problem-focused history requires one to three elements of a review of systems.

99233   A 72-year-old man admitted for depression with suicidal ideation and paranoid delusions is seen for a subsequent hospital visit. The patient is in his seventh hospital day. The attending psychiatrist interviews the patient and does a mental status examination, noting minor changes in orientation. The attending psychiatrist meets with the treatment team and reviews notes prepared by nursing, occupational therapy/recreational therapy, and social work staff. Although the patient is taking antidepressants, the team does not believe the patient has shown progress. His sleep and appetite are poor, and he must be encouraged to shower and groom. The attending psychiatrist reviews discharge planning with social work staff and writes the daily progress note. Later the same day the attending psychiatrist is notified that the patient has become combative with staff and is confused and disoriented. The attending psychiatrist returns to the unit and orders as-needed lorazepam and open-door seclusion. The patient's vital signs are taken, and a modest increase in temperature is observed. The attending psychiatrist orders a medical consultation and an evaluation for the fever and prepares an addendum to the progress note.

Explanation for code choice: The reason the highest level of subsequent hospital care is recommended in this case is the abrupt change in mental state requiring a return to the unit and a detailed evaluation of the situation, with a detailed examination and medical decision making of high complexity. Although the subsequent hospital care codes require only two of the three key components, it is not a bad idea to do a detailed (two to nine elements) review of systems when using these codes.

OFFICE OR OTHER OUTPATIENT CONSULTATIONS

> **Note:** As of January 1, 2010, Medicare does not reimburse for these codes. See Chapter 4 for alternative coding.

99244   A 7-year-old boy referred by his pediatrician is seen in an initial office consultation. The patient was referred because of his short attention span, easy distractibility, and hyperactivity. The history taken during the parents' interview focuses on the patient's family history and psychosocial context, the mother's pregnancy, the patient's early childhood development, and the parents' description of the onset and progression of the symptoms and behaviors. The mental status examination focuses on the patient's affective state, ability to attend and concentrate during the evaluation and observation, and behavior during the session. The patient is scheduled for neuropsychological testing and a return visit with his parents.

Explanation for code choice: The consultation requires a comprehensive history and examination. The medical decision making is moderately complex. Do not forget that a review of systems is required.

99245   An 81-year-old woman referred by her internist is seen in an initial office consultation for evaluation of her mental state. Her family had reported her activity as being markedly decreased and that she was having difficulty maintaining independent self-care. The patient's history reveals that she has congestive heart failure and chronic obstructive pulmonary disease that is in fair control. She had two episodes of depression in her 50s and was treated successfully with antidepressants. The patient reports feelings of general malaise, loss of interest, trouble sleeping, decreased appetite, and problems with memory over a 4-week period. The patient denies awareness of an inability to maintain her home or independent self-care. A mental status examination reveals a poorly groomed, cooperative woman with moderate psychomotor retardation and no speech abnormalities. She appears sad and expresses feelings of depression and has flat affect. Her Mini-Mental State Examination score is 25 of 30 points, with poor recall, attention and concentration deficits, and distortion of figure drawing. A family member is interviewed and confirms most of the history. Neuropsychological testing is ordered, and the patient's case is discussed with the referring physician.

   Explanation for code choice: This case involves mental disorder with significant comorbid medical conditions. The medical decision making is highly complex, supported by a comprehensive history and examination. The history must include a complete review of systems.

INITIAL INPATIENT CONSULTATIONS

> **Note:** As of January 1, 2010, Medicare does not reimburse for these codes. See Chapter 4 for alternative coding.

99253   An initial hospital consultation is provided for a 35-year-old woman referred by obstetrics/gynecology staff after she had a normal vaginal delivery and had asked to talk to a psychiatrist about feelings of depression. A review of her chart reveals an uncomplicated neonatal course and a normal delivery of a healthy baby girl. History taking focuses on symptom onset and progression and the patient's current family/social context. The patient reports that her husband is out of work and is drinking and arguing with her frequently. Two other children are doing well. A mental status examination reveals a cooperative, friendly individual with normal speech, moderately depressed mood (which she relates to her marital stress), full affect, and no psychotic or anxiety symptoms. She is cognitively intact. Her insight is fair, and her judgment is intact. Her desire for marital counseling is supported, and she is given a referral for this service.

   Explanation for code choice: This consultation for a medically stable patient required a detailed history and examination. The medical decision making is of low complexity. The history must include a detailed review of systems (two to nine elements).

99254   An initial hospital consultation is provided for a 19-year-old female referred by department of medicine staff after treatment for ingestion of acetaminophen and alcohol. A review of her chart reveals that symptomatic management was used to treat ingestion of alcohol (her blood alcohol level was 120 mg/dL) and a nonlethal amount of acetaminophen. The patient has no history of medical or surgical problems. History provided by the patient includes a recent breakup with her boyfriend of 3 years, loss of her job, and fighting with her mother. Her family history includes alcohol abuse by the father and two brothers. The patient reports that she has experimented with street drugs, has used alcohol regularly since age 16 years, and has had a history of binge drinking. There is no history of blackouts or delirium tremens. The patient has no current legal problems. A mental status examination reveals a cooperative individual with good eye contact. She asks "When can I get out of here?" and states "I did a stupid thing." The patient is remorseful, and her affect is bright, with a moderate level of depression. She is cognitively intact. She expresses concerns about her boyfriend and states that she probably needs some counseling. She agrees to treatment of alcohol abuse. The patient is cleared for discharge and given a referral to a community psychiatry program for dually diagnosed patients.

Explanation for code choice: The suicide attempt was committed impulsively, and the patient is remorseful and ready for outpatient follow-up. A detailed history and examination are performed, and medical decision making is moderately complex. The history must include a complete review of systems.

99255   An initial hospital consultation is provided for an 82-year-old man referred by department of medicine staff because of bizarre behavior that resulted in his requiring a sitter. The patient has high blood pressure, renal insufficiency, congestive heart failure, and chronic obstructive pulmonary disease. He is taking 12 medications, including as-needed lorazepam and haloperidol for "behavioral control." Notes prepared by nursing staff indicate that the patient has periods of lucidity intermixed with confused, uncooperative behavior, usually in the evenings. The patient began receiving antibiotics in the previous 12 hours for a urinary tract infection. The social worker reports that the patient lives with his wife and was in good health and maintained a wide range of activities before this admission. The wife reports some slippage in the patient's memory, but the patient denies that there are any problems whatsoever. The mental status examination reveals the patient to be resting in his hospital bed and receiving intravenous fluids and intranasal oxygen. The patient is irritable, and his irritability increases during the course of the evaluation. He denies any psychological symptoms. The patient knows who he is and where he is but does not know the day, the date, or the month. He cannot do serial 7s. The patient reports having had a visit by several of his children the night before, but nursing staff report no such visit took place. The findings are reviewed with the nursing staff and the attending physician. Lorazepam is discontinued, and orientation strategies are discussed with the nursing staff and the attending physician.

Explanation for code choice: This case is typical for an acute geriatric medical admission: multiple comorbidities and multiple medications complicated by delirium. The consulting psychiatrist must do a comprehensive history and examination. The medical decision making is highly complex. The history must include a complete review of systems.

Appendix G

Most Frequently Missed Items in Evaluation and Management (E/M) Documentation

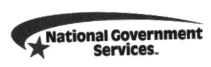
National Government Services, Inc.
1333 Brunswick Avenue
Lawrenceville, New Jersey 08648

A CMS Contracted Agent

Most Frequently Missed Items in Evaluation and Management (E/M) Documentation

History

- History is too brief and lacks the reason for the encounter or minimal documentation of the reason for the encounter.

- Documentation for the Review of Systems is too minimal.

- If billing for a Complete Review of Systems – either must individually document ten (10) or more systems **OR** may document pertinent (some) systems and make the statement in the progress note "all other systems negative."

- Lacks any documentation in support of why elements of the history or the entire history was unobtainable; would also apply to documenting the work done to attempt to obtain history from sources other than the patient if it was unobtainable from the patient.

- Insufficient documentation of the Past, Family and Social history; no reference to dates or any documentation to support obtaining the information.

- If you wish to refer to a Review of Systems and/or a PFSH documented in a progress note of a previous date and update it with today's information (e.g., unchanged from ROS of 1/4/07 except patient has stopped smoking) – you must specifically indicate the previous date you are referring to in today's note and you must include a photocopy of the previous ROS or PFSH you have referred to if you are asked to send documentation for today's note. Make sure your staff is also aware of this if they will photocopy and send documentation to Medicare.

Physical Exam

- Physical exam documentation is too brief.

- 1997 Specialty exams, billed at the comprehensive level, do not meet all of the required elements for that level.

- For the 1995 Comprehensive exam – required to count ONLY organ systems and not body areas; must be eight (8) or more organ systems only.

- Can choose to perform and document either the 1995 or 1997 physical exam but findings show that most physicians do better with documentation based upon the 1995 guidelines.

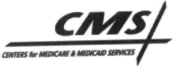

Medical Decision Making

- Lack of sufficient evidence that labs, X-rays, etc., were performed to credit in this section (Amount and/or Complexity of Data Reviewed or in Table of Risk of Complications and/or Morbidity or Mortality).

- Lack of sufficient documentation of items which could be credited to Reviewed Data (Amount and/or Complexity of Data Reviewed) such as the decision to obtain old records or obtain history from someone other than the patient, review and summarization of old records, discussion of case with another health care provider.

- Remember, in this section, need only two (2) elements of the three and need only the highest, single item available and appropriate in one box of the chart for Risk of Complications and/or Morbidity or Mortality.

Time Based Codes

- In choosing a code based upon time for counseling and coordination of care, total time may be documented but there is not quantification that more than 50 percent of the time was spent on counseling and there is also no documentation of what the coordination of care was or what the counseling was.

- No documentation of time for critical care.

- No documentation of time for discharge day management.

General

- Missing the order for a consultation in hospitals and SNFs.

- Illegible documentation.

- Lack of a physician signature on the note.

- Missing patient names.

- Incorrect dates of service.

- Lack of any note for a billed date of service.

- Lack of the required two (2) or three (3) key elements to bill an E/M service.

Appendix H

Documentation Templates

These templates are meant to serve as examples. We recommend that you design and format your own templates using the elements relevant to your practice. Templates can be either paper or electronic.

- Attending Physician Admission Note
- Attending Physician Subsequent Care
- Psychiatric Consultation (see also Chapter 4 for requirements for lower levels of care)
- Attending Consultant Physician Psychiatry Evaluation
- Pharmacologic Management 90862

Attending Physician Admission Note

Note: **Do not forget the review of systems in the attending note for the first day of service**
Initial hospital care 99221–99223
Initial nursing facility care 99304–99306
This template is also appropriate for 90801 (ROS not required)

Patient name: _____

Date: _____

History number: _____

Time: _____

IDENTIFYING INFORMATION AND CHIEF COMPLAINT OR REASON FOR ADMISSION:

FAMILY HISTORY, PERSONAL HISTORY, PREMORBID PERSONALITY:

MEDICAL HISTORY	REVIEW OF SYSTEMS AND ACTIVE MEDICAL PROBLEMS	
Allergies:	Constitutional:	Muscular:
Source of regular care:	Eyes:	Integumentary:
	Ears/Nose/Mouth/Throat:	Neurological:
	Cardiovascular:	Endocrine:
Operation/Injuries:	Respiratory:	Hematologic/Lymphatic:
	Gastrointestinal:	Allergies/Immune:
	Genitourinary:	All others negative:
Diagnoses:	Medications:	

Attending Physician Admission Note *(continued)*

Initial hospital care 99221–99223
Initial nursing facility care 99304–99306
This template is also appropriate for 90801 (ROS not required)

Patient name: _____   Date: _____

History number: _____   Time: _____

PAST PSYCHIATRIC AND
PRESENT ILLNESS:

Informants:	
__ Patient	__ Resident
__ Family	__ Past records
__ Current and past providers	__ Other _____

Elements of history of present illness:
__ Location
__ Quality
__ Severity
__ Duration
__ Timing
__ Content
__ Modifying factors
__ Associated signs and symptoms

Attending Physician Admission Note *(continued)*

Initial hospital care 99221–99223
Initial nursing facility care 99304–99306
This template is also appropriate for 90801 (ROS not required)

Patient name: _____   Date: _____

History number: _____   Time: _____

MENTAL STATUS EXAMINATION

Patient personally examined: __ Yes __ No

Vital signs (3 or more):

Blood pressure: _____ *Supine* / _____ *Sitting* / _____ *Standing*

Pulse: _____ *Regular*   **Respiration:** _____   **Temperature:** _____   **Height:** _____   **Weight:** _____

General appearance and manner	Check (✓) if normal or none: __ Development __ Nutrition __ Habitus __ Deformities __ Grooming
Musculoskeletal (strength/tone/abnormal movements):	Check (✓) if normal or none: __ Strength __ Tone __ Atrophy __ Abnormal movements __ Gait __ Station

Speech (form and processes/content and associations):

Check (✓) if normal:

Speech	Processes	Associations
__ Volume	__ Rate	__ Intact
__ Articulation	__ Logical	
__ Coherence	__ Abstraction	
__ Spontaneity	__ Computation	

Mood and affect:	Check (✓) if none: __ Homicidal ideation __ Suicidal ideation __ Violent ideation
Hallucinations/Delusions:	Check (✓) if none: __ Hallucinations __ Delusions
Anxiety symptoms (obsessions/compulsions/phobias/panic attacks):	Check (✓) if none: __ Obsessions __ Compulsions __ Panic attacks __ Anxiety: __ somatic __ psychic

Attending Physician Admission Note *(continued)*

Initial hospital care 99221–99223
Initial nursing facility care 99304–99306
This template is also appropriate for 90801 (ROS not required)

Patient name: _____   Date: _____

History number: _____   Time: _____

MINI-MENTAL STATE EXAMINATION

Score:

Items missed:

Orientation:

Memory:

Attention/Concentration:

Language:

Fund of knowledge:

Judgment:

Insight:

Other findings:

Check (✔) if normal:
__ Intact

__ Intact

__ Intact

Attending Physician Admission Note *(continued)*

Initial hospital care 99221–99223
Initial nursing facility care 99304–99306
This template is also appropriate for 90801 (ROS not required)

Patient name: _____   Date: _____

History number: _____   Time: _____

MEDICAL DECISION MAKING	
Need for Admission:	**Initial Treatment Plan:**
	Laboratory Tests/Radiology/Tests:
	Consultation:
Medical Records/Laboratory Tests/Data:	Social Work Intervention:
	Discharge Planning:
	Occupational Therapy/Physical Therapy:
Formulation (Diagnoses [use Axes I–V]/Discussion):	Medications:
	Interventions/Therapy:
Observation Status (Rationale): __ Ad lib __ Every-15-minutes checks __ Close observation __ Geri chair __ Open-door seclusion __ Locked-door seclusion __ Other:	

Attending physician name *(print)*

_____   Date

Attending physician signature

From Schmidt CW, Yowell RK, Jaffe E: *Procedure Coding Handbook for Psychiatrists*, 4th Edition.

Attending Physician Subsequent Care (Hospital, Nursing Facility, and Outpatient Established Patient)

Remember—for subsequent hospital and nursing facility care, only two of the three key factors are necessary to meet documentation requirements. Similarly, only two of three key factors are necessary for outpatient office visits for established patients.

Patient Name: _____ Date: _____

History Number: _____ Time: _____

HISTORY AND PROGRESS

History of Present Illness (HPI) **Review of Systems (ROS)** **Other**

Chief Complaint

Neurological:

Sleep   (describe):

1

_____

Headache	__Yes	__No
Weakness	__Yes	__No
Stiffness	__Yes	__No
Tremor	__Yes	__No

2

Gastrointestinal:

Appetite   __Poor   __Fair   __Good

3

Bowel movements (describe):

_____

| Nausea/Vomiting | __Yes | __No |
| Incontinence | __Yes | __No |

Past, Family, and/or Social History (PFSH):

HPI	ROS	PFSH	Level	Inpatient	Nursing Facility
Brief 1–3	NA	NA	Problem focused	99231	99307
Brief 1–3	Problem pertinent (1)	NA	Expanded problem focused	99232	99308
Extended 4+ Comprehensive	Extended (2–9) Complete	Pertinent Comprehensive	Detailed Comprehensive	99233	99309 99310

EXAMINATION

Vital signs (3 or more): **Blood pressure:** _____ *Supine* / _____ *Sitting* / _____ *Standing*

Pulse: _____ *Regular* **Respiration:** _____ **Temperature:** _____ **Weight:** _____

Level of Consciousness: __Alert __Drowsy __Stuporous __Comatose

Orientation: *Person* __Yes __No   *Place* __Yes __No   *Time* __Yes __No | Attention/Concentration

Memory: *Recent:*   *Remote:*

Speech: *Rate:*   *Rhythm:*   *Volume:*   Pressured __Yes __No

Thought Processes: | **Associations:**

Mood: | **Expressed Emotion/Affect:** | **Range of Affect:**

Self Attitude:

Passive death wish __Yes __No   Suicidal thoughts: __Yes __No   Homicidal thoughts: __Yes __No

Perceptual Phenomena: | **Ideational Phenomena:**

Hallucinations: __Yes __No   *Illusions:* __Yes __No   *Delusions:* __Yes __No

__Auditory __Visual __Tactile   Content: Content:

__Olfactory __Gustatory __Visceral   *Obsessions:* __Yes __No
Content:

From Schmidt CW, Yowell RK, Jaffe E: *Procedure Coding Handbook for Psychiatrists*, 4th Edition.
Copyright © 2011 American Psychiatric Association (www.appi.org)

Attending Physician Subsequent Care (Hospital, Nursing Facility, and Outpatient Established Patient) *(continued)*

Patient Name: _____   Date: _____

History Number: _____   Time: _____

Fund of Knowledge: Insight: __Poor __Fair __Good Judgment __Poor __Fair __Good

Strength:

Tone: __Normal
      __Increased
      __Decreased

Gate:

Station:

Abnormal Movements:
__None
__Tremor
__Oral dyskinesia
__Choreoathetosis
__Other:_____

Level	Examination elements
Problem focused	1–5
Expanded	6
Detailed	9

Attending Physician Subsequent Care (Hospital, Nursing Facility, and Outpatient Established Patient) *(continued)*

Patient Name: _____   Date: _____

History Number: _____   Time: _____

MEDICAL DECISION MAKING

Problem/Condition: __New __Established	**Status:** __Improving __Worsening	**Comorbidities:** __Stable __Complications/side effects __Independent management required __Interference with management of primary condition(s)

Formulation (Diagnostic/Decision/Rationale for Continuing Hospitalization):

Treatment Plans:

Medical Records/Laboratory Tests/Consultations:

Observation Status (Rationale):
__Ad lib
__Every-15-minutes checks
__Close observation
__Geri chair
__Open-door seclusion
__Locked-door seclusion
__Other:

_____

Attending consultant physician name *(print)*

_____

Attending consultant physician signature   Date

Psychiatric Consultation (inpatient 99255 or outpatient 99245 when fully completed)

Medicare no longer pays for the consultation codes. When coding for Medicare or for commercial carriers that have followed Medicare's lead, 90801 may be used for both inpatient and outpatient consults. Psychiatrists who choose to use E/M codes to report outpatient consults should use the outpatient new patient codes (99201–99205). For inpatient consults, the codes to use are hospital inpatient services, initial hospital care for new or established patients (99221–99223). For consults in nursing homes, initial nursing facility care codes should be used (99304–99306); if the consult is of low complexity, the subsequent nursing facility codes may be used (99307–99310). As with all E/M codes, the selection of the specific code is based on the complexity of the case and the amount of work required. Medicare has created a new modifier, A1, to denote the admitting physician so that more than one physician may use the initial hospital care codes.

Patient name: _____ Date: _____

History number: _____ Time: _____

IDENTIFYING INFORMATION AND CHIEF COMPLAINT:

FAMILY HISTORY, PERSONAL HISTORY, PREMORBID PERSONALITY:

Family history:
__ Family diseases/traits and treatment
__ Deaths/Suicides in family

Social history:
__ Alcohol use	__ Marital status
__ Tobacco use	__ Living conditions
__ Illicit drug use	__ Education
__ Sexual history	__ Employment

MEDICAL HISTORY	REVIEW OF SYSTEMS AND ACTIVE MEDICAL PROBLEMS	
Allergies:	Constitutional:	Muscular:
Source of regular care:	Eyes:	Integumentary:
Operation/Injuries:	Ears/Nose/Mouth/Throat:	Neurological:
Prior hospitalizations:	Cardiovascular:	Endocrine:
	Respiratory:	Hematologic/Lymphatic:
Diagnoses:	Gastrointestinal:	Allergies/Immune:
	Genitourinary:	All others negative:
	Reference to chart: _____ (date)	
Medications:	**PHYSICAL EXAMINATION**	
	Reference to chart: _____ (date)	

From Schmidt CW, Yowell RK, Jaffe E: *Procedure Coding Handbook for Psychiatrists*, 4th Edition.
Copyright © 2011 American Psychiatric Association (www.appi.org)

Attending Consultant Physician Psychiatry Evaluation

The consultation template is an example of a comprehensive level of care (99245 or 99255) if fully completed. All levels of consultations require a review of systems to varying degrees of completion (see Chapter 4 for requirements).

Patient name: _____   Date: _____

History number: _____   Time: _____

HISTORY OF PRESENT ILLNESS:

Informants:

__ Patient   __ Resident

__ Family   __ Past records

__ Current and past providers   __ Other _____

Elements of history of present illness:

__ Location

__ Quality

__ Severity

__ Duration

__ Timing

__ Content

__ Modifying factors

__ Associated signs and symptoms

PAST PSYCHIATRIC HISTORY:

From Schmidt CW, Yowell RK, Jaffe E: *Procedure Coding Handbook for Psychiatrists*, 4th Edition.

Attending Consultant Physician Psychiatry Evaluation *(continued)*

Patient name: _____ Date: _____

History number: _____ Time: _____

MENTAL STATUS EXAMINATION

Patient personally examined: __ Yes __ No

Vital signs (3 or more): Vitals reviewed from chart: _____ (date)

Blood pressure: _____ *Supine* / _____ *Sitting* / _____ *Standing*

Pulse: _____ *Regular* **Respiration:** _____ **Temperature:** _____ **Weight:** _____

General appearance and manner:	Check (✔) if normal or none: __ Development __ Nutrition __ Habitus __ Deformities __ Grooming
Musculoskeletal (strength/tone/abnormal movements):	Check (✔) if normal or none: __ Strength __ Tone __ Atrophy __ Abnormal movements __ Gait __ Station

Speech (form and processes/content and associations):

Check (✔) if normal:

Speech	Processes	Associations
__ Volume	__ Rate	__ Intact
__ Articulation	__ Logical	
__ Coherence	__ Abstraction	
__ Spontaneity	__ Computation	

Mood and affect:	Check (✔) if none: __ Homicidal ideation __ Suicidal ideation __ Violent ideation
Hallucinations/Delusions:	Check (✔) if none: __ Hallucinations __ Delusions
Anxiety symptoms (obsessions/compulsions/phobias/panic attacks):	Check (✔) if none: __ Obsessions __ Compulsions __ Panic attacks __ Anxiety: __ somatic __ psychic

Attending Consultant Physician Psychiatry Evaluation *(continued)*

Patient name: _____   Date: _____

History number: _____   Time: _____

MINI-MENTAL STATE EXAMINATION

Score:

Items missed:

Orientation:

Memory:

Attention/Concentration:

Language:

Fund of knowledge:

Judgment:

Insight:

Check (✓) if normal:
__ Intact

__ Intact

__ Intact

LABORATORY TESTS/DIAGNOSTIC STUDIES

Attending Consultant Physician Psychiatry Evaluation *(continued)*

Patient name: _____   Date: _____

History number: _____   Time: _____

MEDICAL DECISION MAKING
Diagnoses:

Axis I:

Axis II:

Axis III:

Axis IV:

Axis V:

Discussed with:
__ Attending
__ House staff
__ Family
__ Outside physician
__ Care provider

RECOMMENDATIONS:

Diagnostic:

Therapeutic:

Attending consultant physician name *(print)*

Attending consultant physician signature   Date

From Schmidt CW, Yowell RK, Jaffe E: *Procedure Coding Handbook for Psychiatrists*, 4th Edition.
Copyright © 2011 American Psychiatric Association (www.appi.org)

Pharmacologic Management 90862

Patient name: _____   Date: _____ _____

History number: _____   Time: _____

Length of face-to-face service: _____
(usually at least 15 minutes face-to-face)

Interval history:

Mental status exam:

Response to medications and assessment of side effects:

Laboratory tests reviewed:

Laboratory tests ordered:

Diagnoses:

Legible signature

ECT Patient Information, Consent Form, and Record Template

ECT PATIENT INFORMATION

My doctor has recommended that I receive treatment with electroconvulsive therapy (ECT).

I understand that there may be other treatments for my condition, including medications and psychotherapy, and that whether ECT or another treatment is more appropriate depends on a person's prior experience with these treatments, the nature of his/her psychiatric condition, and other considerations. My doctor has explained to me why ECT has been recommended for my specific case.

The potential benefit of ECT for me is that it may lead to improvement in my psychiatric condition. ECT has been shown to be a highly effective treatment for a number of conditions. However, not all patients respond equally well. As with all forms of medical treatment, some patients recover quickly; others recover only to relapse again and require further treatment; while still others fail to respond at all. Very rarely a switch into the manic phase of manic-depressive illness can occur.

Procedure

ECT involves a series of treatments. For each treatment, I will be brought to a specially equipped room in this hospital. The treatments are usually given in the morning, before breakfast. Because the treatments involve general anesthesia,

---

From Schmidt CW, Yowell RK, Jaffe E: *Procedure Coding Handbook for Psychiatrists,* Fourth Edition. Copyright © 2011 American Psychiatric Association (www.appi.org).

I will have had nothing to drink or eat for at least 6 hours before each treatment, unless special orders have been written by my doctor for me to receive medicines with a sip of water. An intravenous line will be placed so that I can be given medications as part of the procedure. One of these will be an anesthetic drug that will quickly put me to sleep. When I am asleep, I will be given a second drug that will relax my muscles. Because I will be asleep, I will not experience pain or discomfort during the procedure. I will not feel the electrical current, and when I wake up I will have no memory of the treatment.

To prepare for the treatments, monitoring sensors will be placed on my head and chest. Blood pressure cuffs will be placed on one arm and one ankle. This will enable the physician to monitor my brain waves, my heart, and my blood pressure. These recordings involve no pain or discomfort.

After I am asleep, a small, carefully controlled amount of electricity will be passed between two electrodes that have been placed on my head. Depending on where the electrodes are placed, I may receive either bilateral ECT or unilateral ECT. In bilateral ECT, one electrode is placed on the left side of the head, the other is on the right side. In unilateral ECT, both electrodes are placed on the same side of the head, usually on the right side. When the current is passed, a generalized seizure is produced in the brain. Because I will have been given a medication to relax my muscles, muscular contractions in my body that would ordinarily accompany a seizure will be considerably softened. I will be given oxygen to breathe. The seizure will last for approximately 1 minute.

Recovery

Within a few minutes, the anesthetic drug will wear off and I will awaken. I will be in a recovery room, where I will be observed until I am ready to leave the ECT area.

Number of Treatments

The number of treatments that I will receive cannot be predicted ahead of time. The number of treatments will depend on my psychiatric condition, how quickly I respond to the treatment, and the medical judgment of my psychiatrist. Typically, 6 to 12 treatments are given. However, some patients respond slowly and more treatments may be required. Treatments are usually given three times a week, but the frequency of treatment may also vary depending on my needs.

Risks

As with all forms of medical treatment, there is a possibility of some side effects of treatment. I may have a headache, muscle soreness, or nausea. These side effects usually respond to simple treatment. Minor irregularities in heart rate and rhythm often occur. Very rarely, myocardial infarction (heart attack) or stroke can occur. Dislocations or bone fracture, and dental complications occur extremely rarely. As with any general anesthetic procedure, there is a remote possibility of death. It is estimated that fatality associated with ECT occurs in approximately 1 per 10,000 patients treated.

To reduce the risk of medical complications, I will receive a careful medical evaluation prior to starting ECT.

However, despite precautions there is a small chance that I will experience a medical complication. Should this occur, I understand that medical care and treatment are available. I understand, however, that neither the institution nor the treating physicians are required to provide long-term medical treatment. I shall be responsible for the cost of such treatment whether personally or through medical insurance or other medical coverage. I understand that no compensation will be paid for lost wages or other consequential damages.

Memory Problems

Memory difficulties are common just after treatment. As time passes following treatment, memory functioning improves. Shortly after the course of ECT, I may experience difficulties remembering events that happened before and while I receive ECT. Gaps in memory for past events may extend back to several months before I received ECT, and in rare instances, up to 1 or 2 years. Many of these memories will return during the first several months following the ECT course.

In addition, for a short period following ECT, I may experience difficulty in learning and remembering new information. This difficulty in forming new memories, if it occurs, should be temporary and will most likely subside within several weeks following the ECT course.

Individuals vary considerably in the extent to which they experience confusion and memory problems during and shortly following treatment with ECT. Many patients actually report that their learning and memory functioning is improved after ECT compared to their functioning prior to the treatment course.

A small minority of patients, perhaps 1 in 200, report severe problems in memory that remain for months or even years. The reasons for these rare reports of long-lasting impairment are not fully understood. I may be left with some permanent gaps in my memory, particularly for events occurring close to the ECT treatment.

Right unilateral ECT (electrodes on the right side) produces less memory impairment than bilateral ECT (one electrode on each side of the head).

Because of the possible problems with confusion and memory, it is important that I not make any important personal or business decisions during the ECT course. This may mean postponing decisions regarding financial or family matters. After the treatment course, I will begin a "convalescence period," usually 1 to 3 weeks, but which varies from patient to patient. During this period I should refrain from driving, transacting business, or other activities for which impairment of memory may be problematic until I am advised by my doctor that I am ready to do these things.

Further Questions

I understand that I should feel free to ask my doctor or any other member of the ECT treatment team questions about ECT at this time or at any time during the ECT course or thereafter. I also understand that my decision to agree to ECT is being made on a voluntary basis and that I may withdraw my consent and have the treatments stopped at any time.

ECT Consent Form

I, the undersigned, understand the hazards and potential dangers involved in treatment by means of electroconvulsive therapy. I acknowledge that Dr. _____
has explained the purpose of the procedure, the anesthesia, the risk involved, alternatives, and the possibility of complications. I have read the preceding information or it has been read to me, and all my questions regarding this procedure have been answered to my satisfaction.

I hereby give my consent and authorize and request the staff of _____ to give electroconvulsive therapy to _____ and if during the treatment other conditions arise which, in the best judgment of the medical staff, require emergency treatment, I authorize and request that the said treatment be performed. I further understand that no guarantee of any results has been made.

I consent to the admission of medical students and other authorized observers during the treatment, in accordance with ordinary practices of this hospital.

I have read carefully, and I understand, the foregoing.

Patient's Signature: _____

Witness: _____

Date: _____   Time: _____

I have carefully read and understand the foregoing, and I join in consenting to the performance upon the above patient of the treatment referred to above.

Relative or Guardian: _____

Witness: _____

Date: _____   Time: _____

ECT Record

DATE	TX NUMBER	ELECTRODE PLACEMENT	PULSE WIDTH	PULSE FREQUENCY	STIMULUS DURATION	CURRENT	SEIZURE DURATION	COMMENTS	ATTENDING PHYSICIAN SIGNATURE AND PRINTED NAME
									Signature _____ _Print name_ _____
									Signature _____ _Print name_ _____
									Signature _____ _Print name_ _____
									Signature _____ _Print name_ _____
									Signature _____ _Print name_ _____

Appendix J

Examples of Relative Value Units (RVUs) (2010)

Note: The conversion factor in January 2010 was 36.0846. Fees provided in this chart have been calculated using the following formula: ([Work RVU] + [Practice Expense RVU] + [Malpractice RVU]) x Conversion Factor = Fee. The amounts listed may not reflect the exact amount you will receive for your services because further adjustments based on variables such as geographic location may be made. Fees for your specific locale can be found on your Medicare contractor's Web site.

2010 NATIONAL MEDICARE PHYSICIAN FEE SCHEDULE: RELATIVE VALUE UNITS (RVUs) AND FEES

CPT CODE	DESCRIPTION	WORK RVU	NON-FACILITY PE RVU	FACILITY PE RVU	MP RVU	NON-FACILITY TOTAL	FACILITY TOTAL	NON-FACILITY FEE	FACILITY FEE
90801	Psychiatric diagnostic interview	2.80	1.38	0.65	0.08	4.26	3.53	$153.72	$127.38
90802	Intac psychiatric diagnostic interview	3.01	1.47	0.71	0.10	4.58	3.82	$165.27	$137.84
90804	Psytx, office, 20–30 min	1.21	0.52	0.24	0.03	1.76	1.48	$63.51	$53.41
90805	Psytx, office, 20–30 min with E/M	1.37	0.58	0.28	0.04	1.99	1.69	$71.81	$60.98
90806	Psytx, office, 45–50 min	1.86	0.53	0.36	0.05	2.44	2.27	$88.05	$81.91
90807	Psytx, office, 45–50 min with E/M	2.02	0.71	0.41	0.06	2.79	2.49	$100.68	$89.85
90808	Psytx, office, 75–80 min	2.79	0.72	0.54	0.08	3.59	3.41	$129.54	$123.05
90809	Psytx, office, 75–80 min with E/M	2.95	0.90	0.62	0.10	3.95	3.67	$142.53	$132.43
90810	Intac psytx, office, 20–30 min	1.32	0.51	0.26	0.04	1.87	1.62	$67.48	$58.46
90811	Intac psytx, 20–30 min with E/M	1.48	0.69	0.31	0.05	2.22	1.84	$80.11	$66.40
90812	Intac psytx, office, 45–50 min	1.97	0.64	0.38	0.05	2.66	2.40	$95.99	$86.60
90813	Intac psytx, 45–50 min with E/M	2.13	0.82	0.44	0.07	3.02	2.64	$108.98	$95.26
90814	Intac psytx, office, 75–80 min	2.90	0.88	0.62	0.09	3.87	3.61	$139.65	$130.27
90815	Intac psytx, 75–80 min with E/M	3.06	1.02	0.64	0.10	4.18	3.80	$150.83	$137.12
90816	Psytx, hospital, 20–30 min	1.25	0.33	0.33	0.03	1.61	1.61	$58.10	$58.10
90817	Psytx, hospital, 20–30 min with E/M	1.41	0.38	0.38	0.05	1.84	1.84	$66.40	$66.40
90818	Psytx, hospital, 45–50 min	1.89	0.46	0.46	0.05	2.40	2.40	$86.60	$86.60
90819	Psytx, hospital, 45–50 min with E/M	2.05	0.51	0.51	0.07	2.63	2.63	$94.90	$94.90
90821	Psytx, hospital, 75–80 min	2.83	0.64	0.64	0.08	3.55	3.55	$128.10	$128.10
90822	Psytx, hospital, 75–80 min with E/M	2.99	0.70	0.70	0.10	3.79	3.79	$136.76	$136.76
90823	Intac psytx, hospital, 20–30 min	1.36	0.34	0.34	0.04	1.74	1.74	$62.79	$62.79
90824	Intac psytx, hospital, 20–30 min with E/M	1.52	0.40	0.40	0.05	1.97	1.97	$71.09	$71.09
90826	Intac psytx, hospital, 45–50 min	2.01	0.48	0.48	0.05	2.54	2.54	$91.65	$91.65
90827	Intac psytx, hospital, 45–50 min with E/M	2.16	0.53	0.53	0.07	2.76	2.76	$99.59	$99.59

2010 NATIONAL MEDICARE PHYSICIAN FEE SCHEDULE: RELATIVE VALUE UNITS (RVUs) AND FEES (CONTINUED)

CPT CODE	DESCRIPTION	WORK RVU	NON-FACILITY PE RVU	FACILITY PE RVU	MP RVU	NON-FACILITY TOTAL	FACILITY TOTAL	NON-FACILITY FEE	FACILITY FEE
90828	Intac psytx, hospital, 75–80 min	2.94	0.66	0.66	0.08	3.68	3.68	$132.79	$132.79
90829	Intac psytx, hospital, 75–80 min with E/M	3.10	0.72	0.72	0.10	3.92	3.92	$141.45	$141.45
90845	Psychoanalysis	1.79	0.43	0.38	0.05	2.27	2.22	$81.91	$80.11
90846	Family psytx without patient	1.83	0.52	0.46	0.05	2.40	2.34	$86.60	$84.44
90847	Family psytx with patient	2.21	0.72	0.53	0.06	2.99	2.80	$107.89	$101.04
90849	Multiple family group psytx	0.59	0.30	0.21	0.02	0.91	0.82	$32.84	$29.59
90853	Group psychotherapy	0.59	0.27	0.21	0.02	0.88	0.82	$31.75	$29.59
90857	Intac group psytx	0.63	0.33	0.22	0.02	0.98	0.87	$35.36	$31.39
90862	Medication management	0.95	0.58	0.28	0.03	1.56	1.26	$56.29	$45.47
90865	Narcosynthesis	2.84	1.38	0.70	0.09	4.31	3.63	$155.52	$130.99
90870	Electroconvulsive therapy	1.88	1.90	0.43	0.06	3.84	2.37	$138.56	$85.52
90875	Psychophysiological therapy	1.20	0.74	0.43	0.06	2.00	1.69	$72.17	$60.98
90876	Psychophysiological therapy	1.90	0.97	0.68	0.10	2.97	2.68	$107.17	$96.71
90880	Hypnotherapy	2.19	0.64	0.44	0.06	2.89	2.69	$104.28	$97.07
90882	Environmental manipulation	0.00	0.00	0.00	0.00	0.00	0.00	$0.00	$0.00
90885	Psychiatric evaluation of records	0.97	0.35	0.35	0.05	1.37	1.37	$49.44	$49.44
90887	Consultation with family	1.48	0.82	0.53	0.07	2.37	2.08	$85.52	$75.06
90889	Preparation of report	0.00	0.00	0.00	0.00	0.00	0.00	$0.00	$0.00
90899	Psychiatric service/therapy	0.00	0.00	0.00	0.00	0.00	0.00	$0.00	$0.00
90901	Biofeedback training, any method	0.41	0.52	0.12	0.02	0.95	0.55	$34.28	$19.85
90911	Biofeedback peri/uro/rectal	0.89	1.40	0.32	0.05	2.34	1.26	$84.44	$45.47
90935	Hemodialysis, one evaluation	1.22	0.60	0.60	0.05	1.87	1.87	$67.48	$67.48
90937	Hemodialysis, repeated evaluations	2.11	0.88	0.88	0.09	3.08	3.08	$111.14	$111.14
90940	Hemodialysis access study	0.00	0.00	0.00	0.00	0.00	0.00	$0.00	$0.00

2010 National Medicare Physician Fee Schedule: Relative Value Units (RVUs) and Fees (continued)

CPT CODE	DESCRIPTION	WORK RVU	NON-FACILITY PE RVU	FACILITY PE RVU	MP RVU	NON-FACILITY TOTAL	FACILITY TOTAL	NON-FACILITY FEE	FACILITY FEE
96101	Psychological testing by psychiatrist/physician	1.86	0.39	0.38	0.05	2.30	2.29	$82.99	$82.63
96102	Psychological testing by technician	0.50	0.94	0.12	0.03	1.47	0.65	$53.04	$23.45
96103	Psychological testing administered by computer	0.51	0.85	0.14	0.02	1.38	0.67	$49.80	$24.18
96105	Assessment of aphasia	0.00	2.04	2.04	0.03	2.07	2.07	$74.70	$74.70
96110	Developmental test, limited	0.00	0.19	0.19	0.01	0.20	0.20	$7.22	$7.22
96111	Developmental test, extended	2.60	0.89	0.79	0.12	3.61	3.51	$130.27	$126.66
96116	Neurobehavioral status examination	1.86	0.61	0.47	0.07	2.54	2.40	$91.65	$86.60
96118	Neuropsychiatric testing by psychiatrist/physician	1.86	0.88	0.37	0.05	2.79	2.28	$100.68	$82.27
96119	Neuropsychiatric testing by technician	0.55	1.31	0.12	0.02	1.88	0.69	$67.84	$24.90
96120	Neuropsychiatric testing administered by computer	0.51	1.49	0.13	0.02	2.02	0.66	$72.89	$23.82
96125	Cognitive test by hc pro	1.70	0.85	0.45	0.05	2.60	2.20	$93.82	$79.39
96150	Assess health/behavior, initial	0.50	0.11	0.10	0.01	0.62	0.61	$22.37	$22.01
96151	Assess health/behavior, subsequent	0.48	0.11	0.10	0.01	0.60	0.59	$21.65	$21.29
96152	Intervene health/behavior, individual	0.46	0.10	0.09	0.01	0.57	0.56	$20.57	$20.21
96153	Intervene health/behavior, group	0.10	0.03	0.02	0.01	0.14	0.13	$5.05	$4.69
96154	Intervene health/behavior, family with patient	0.45	0.10	0.09	0.01	0.56	0.55	$20.21	$19.85
96155	Intervene health/behavior, family without patient	0.44	0.16	0.16	0.02	0.62	0.62	$22.37	$22.37
99201	Office/Outpatient visit, new	0.48	0.57	0.18	0.03	1.08	0.69	$38.97	$24.90
99202	Office/Outpatient visit, new	0.93	0.88	0.35	0.06	1.87	1.34	$67.48	$48.35
99203	Office/Outpatient visit, new	1.42	1.19	0.50	0.10	2.71	2.02	$97.79	$72.89
99204	Office/Outpatient visit, new	2.43	1.61	0.82	0.16	4.20	3.41	$151.56	$123.05
99205	Office/Outpatient visit, new	3.17	1.91	1.05	0.20	5.28	4.42	$190.53	$159.49

2010 NATIONAL MEDICARE PHYSICIAN FEE SCHEDULE: RELATIVE VALUE UNITS (RVUs) AND FEES (CONTINUED)

CPT CODE	DESCRIPTION	WORK RVU	NON-FACILITY PE RVU	FACILITY PE RVU	MP RVU	NON-FACILITY TOTAL	FACILITY TOTAL	NON-FACILITY FEE	FACILITY FEE
99211	Office/Outpatient visit, established	0.18	0.34	0.06	0.01	0.53	0.25	$19.12	$9.02
99212	Office/Outpatient visit, established	0.48	0.57	0.17	0.03	1.08	0.68	$38.97	$24.54
99213	Office/Outpatient visit, established	0.97	0.80	0.32	0.05	1.82	1.34	$65.67	$48.35
99214	Office/Outpatient visit, established	1.50	1.15	0.49	0.08	2.73	2.07	$98.51	$74.70
99215	Office/Outpatient visit, established	2.11	1.46	0.70	0.11	3.68	2.92	$132.79	$105.37
99217	Observation care discharge	1.28	0.54	0.54	0.06	1.88	1.88	NA	$67.84
99218	Observation care	1.28	0.42	0.42	0.07	1.77	1.77	NA	$63.87
99219	Observation care	2.14	0.69	0.69	0.10	2.93	2.93	NA	$105.73
99220	Observation care	2.99	0.97	0.97	0.14	4.10	4.10	NA	$147.95
99221	Initial hospital care	1.92	0.59	0.59	0.13	2.64	2.64	NA	$95.26
99222	Initial hospital care	2.61	0.82	0.82	0.15	3.58	3.58	NA	$129.18
99223	Initial hospital care	3.86	1.20	1.20	0.20	5.26	5.26	NA	$189.80
99231	Subsequent hospital care	0.76	0.26	0.26	0.04	1.06	1.06	NA	$38.25
99232	Subsequent hospital care	1.39	0.45	0.45	0.07	1.91	1.91	NA	$68.92
99233	Subsequent hospital care	2.00	0.64	0.64	0.10	2.74	2.74	NA	$98.87
99234	Observation/Hospital same date	2.56	0.88	0.88	0.15	3.59	3.59	NA	$129.54
99235	Observation/Hospital same date	3.41	1.13	1.13	0.17	4.71	4.71	NA	$169.96
99236	Observation/Hospital same date	4.26	1.38	1.38	0.20	5.84	5.84	NA	$210.73
99238	Hospital discharge day	1.28	0.54	0.54	0.06	1.88	1.88	NA	$67.84
99239	Hospital discharge day	1.90	0.76	0.76	0.08	2.74	2.74	NA	$98.87
99241	Office consultation	0.64	0.66	0.24	0.05	1.35	0.93	$48.71	$33.56
99242	Office consultation	1.34	1.10	0.51	0.10	2.54	1.95	$91.65	$70.36
99243	Office consultation	1.88	1.46	0.71	0.13	3.47	2.72	$125.21	$98.15
99244	Office consultation	3.02	1.96	1.14	0.16	5.14	4.32	$185.47	$155.89
99245	Office consultation	3.77	2.30	1.38	0.21	6.28	5.36	$226.61	$193.41

2010 National Medicare Physician Fee Schedule: Relative Value Units (RVUs) and Fees (*CONTINUED*)

CPT CODE	DESCRIPTION	WORK RVU	NON-FACILITY PE RVU	FACILITY PE RVU	MP RVU	NON-FACILITY TOTAL	FACILITY TOTAL	NON-FACILITY FEE	FACILITY FEE
99251	Inpatient consultation	1.00	0.32	0.32	0.05	1.37	1.37	NA	$49.44
99252	Inpatient consultation	1.50	0.52	0.52	0.09	2.11	2.11	NA	$76.14
99253	Inpatient consultation	2.27	0.84	0.84	0.11	3.22	3.22	NA	$116.19
99254	Inpatient consultation	3.29	1.23	1.23	0.13	4.65	4.65	NA	$167.79
99255	Inpatient consultation	4.00	1.44	1.44	0.18	5.62	5.62	NA	$202.80
99281	Emergency department visit	0.45	0.10	0.10	0.03	0.58	0.58	NA	$20.93
99282	Emergency department visit	0.88	0.19	0.19	0.05	1.12	1.12	NA	$40.41
99283	Emergency department visit	1.34	0.29	0.29	0.08	1.71	1.71	NA	$61.70
99284	Emergency department visit	2.56	0.50	0.50	0.15	3.21	3.21	NA	$115.83
99285	Emergency department visit	3.80	0.72	0.72	0.22	4.74	4.74	NA	$171.04
99288	Direct advanced life support	0.00	0.00	0.00	0.00	0.00	0.00	NA	$0.00
99291	Critical care, first hour	4.50	2.41	1.24	0.25	7.16	5.99	$258.37	$216.15
99292	Critical care, additional 30 min	2.25	0.86	0.62	0.12	3.23	2.99	$116.55	$107.89
99304	Nursing facility care, initial	1.64	0.62	0.62	0.10	2.36	2.36	$85.16	$85.16
99305	Nursing facility care, initial	2.35	0.82	0.82	0.14	3.31	3.31	$119.44	$119.44
99306	Nursing facility care, initial	3.06	1.01	1.01	0.16	4.23	4.23	$152.64	$152.64
99307	Nursing facility care, subsequent	0.76	0.34	0.34	0.03	1.13	1.13	$40.78	$40.78
99308	Nursing facility care, subsequent	1.16	0.53	0.53	0.05	1.74	1.74	$62.79	$62.79
99309	Nursing facility care, subsequent	1.55	0.68	0.68	0.07	2.30	2.30	$82.99	$82.99
99310	Nursing facility care, subsequent	2.35	0.95	0.95	0.10	3.40	3.40	$122.69	$122.69
99315	Nursing facility discharge day	1.13	0.47	0.47	0.05	1.65	1.65	$59.54	$59.54
99316	Nursing facility discharge day	1.50	0.59	0.59	0.07	2.16	2.16	$77.94	$77.94
99318	Annual nursing facility assessment	1.71	0.63	0.63	0.07	2.41	2.41	$86.96	$86.96

Examples of Relative Value Units (RVUs) (2010)

2010 NATIONAL MEDICARE PHYSICIAN FEE SCHEDULE: RELATIVE VALUE UNITS (RVUs) AND FEES (CONTINUED)

CPT CODE	DESCRIPTION	WORK RVU	NON-FACILITY PE RVU	FACILITY PE RVU	MP RVU	NON-FACILITY TOTAL	FACILITY TOTAL	NON-FACILITY FEE	FACILITY FEE
99324	Domicile/R-home visit, new patient	1.01	0.45	0.45	0.05	1.51	1.51	$54.49	$54.49
99325	Domicile/R-home visit, new patient	1.52	0.60	0.60	0.08	2.20	2.20	$79.39	$79.39
99326	Domicile/R-home visit, new patient	2.63	0.94	0.94	0.12	3.69	3.69	$133.15	$133.15
99327	Domicile/R-home visit, new patient	3.46	1.20	1.20	0.15	4.81	4.81	$173.57	$173.57
99328	Domicile/R-home visit, new patient	4.09	1.38	1.38	0.17	5.64	5.64	$203.52	$203.52
99334	Domicile/R-home visit, established patient	1.07	0.46	0.46	0.05	1.58	1.58	$57.01	$57.01
99335	Domicile/R-home visit, established patient	1.72	0.66	0.66	0.08	2.46	2.46	$88.77	$88.77
99336	Domicile/R-home visit, established patient	2.46	0.89	0.89	0.11	3.46	3.46	$124.85	$124.85
99337	Domicile/R-home visit, established patient	3.58	1.23	1.23	0.16	4.97	4.97	$179.34	$179.34
99339	Domicile/R-home care supervis	1.25	0.76	0.76	0.06	2.07	2.07	$74.70	$74.70
99340	Domicile/r-home care supervis	1.80	1.02	1.02	0.09	2.91	2.91	$105.01	$105.01
99341	Home visit, new patient	1.01	0.45	0.45	0.06	1.52	1.52	$54.85	$54.85
99342	Home visit, new patient	1.52	0.59	0.59	0.08	2.19	2.19	$79.03	$79.03
99343	Home visit, new patient	2.53	0.91	0.91	0.13	3.57	3.57	$128.82	$128.82
99344	Home visit, new patient	3.38	1.19	1.19	0.15	4.72	4.72	$170.32	$170.32
99345	Home visit, new patient	4.09	1.41	1.41	0.18	5.68	5.68	$204.96	$204.96
99347	Home visit, established patient	1.00	0.44	0.44	0.05	1.49	1.49	$53.77	$53.77
99348	Home visit, established patient	1.56	0.61	0.61	0.08	2.25	2.25	$81.19	$81.19
99349	Home visit, established patient	2.33	0.86	0.86	0.11	3.30	3.30	$119.08	$119.08
99350	Home visit, established patient	3.28	1.16	1.16	0.14	4.58	4.58	$165.27	$165.27
99354	Prolonged service, office	1.77	0.74	0.60	0.08	2.59	2.45	$93.46	$88.41
99355	Prolonged service, office	1.77	0.72	0.57	0.09	2.58	2.43	$93.10	$87.69
99356	Prolonged service, inpatient	1.71	0.59	0.59	0.08	2.38	2.38	$85.88	$85.88
99357	Prolonged service, inpatient	1.71	0.59	0.59	0.08	2.38	2.38	NA	$85.88
99358	Prolonged service without contact	2.10	0.77	0.77	0.11	2.98	2.98	$107.53	$107.53

Note.   CPT = Current Procedural Terminology; E/M = evaluation and management; MP = malpractice; PE = practice expense.

Appendix K

National Distribution of Evaluation and Management Code Selection by Psychiatrists

The following table shows the frequency with which psychiatrists used a particular evaluation and management (E/M) code from within a family of E/M codes. For example, psychiatrists billed Current Procedural Terminology (CPT) code 99232 46.55% of the time when providing subsequent hospital care. For comparison purposes we have included data from 2001, 2006, and 2007.

NATIONAL DISTRIBUTION OF EVALUATION AND MANAGEMENT CODE SELECTION BY PSYCHIATRISTS

CODE	NATIONAL DISTRIBUTION 2001, %	NATIONAL DISTRIBUTION 2006, %	NATIONAL DISTRIBUTION 2007, %	NATIONAL DISTRIBUTION 2008, %
Office/Outpatient visits, new patient				
99201	2.01	3.51	1.59	1.59
99202	4.84	4.57	4.67	4.30
99203	19.25	18.59	16.57	15.94
99204	29.67	29.17	24.79	23.90
99205	44.23	44.17	52.38	54.28
Office/Outpatient visits, established patient				
99211	20.96	17.07	13.72	12.42
99212	9.36	5.75	4.86	4.29
99213	29.50	24.09	25.54	23.61
99214	29.04	39.57	38.76	41.27
99215	11.14	13.52	17.13	18.41
Observation care				
99218	30.21	24.77	25.92	19.30
99219	41.73	55.86	43.97	50.01
99220	28.06	19.38	30.11	30.69
Initial hospital care				
99221	11.92	11.85	11.59	11.28
99222	36.53	38.53	37.83	37.52
99223	51.54	49.61	50.58	51.20

NATIONAL DISTRIBUTION OF EVALUATION AND MANAGEMENT CODE SELECTION BY PSYCHIATRISTS (CONTINUED)

CODE	NATIONAL DISTRIBUTION 2001, %	NATIONAL DISTRIBUTION 2006, %	NATIONAL DISTRIBUTION 2007, %	NATIONAL DISTRIBUTION 2008, %
Subsequent hospital care				
99231	43.93	36.08	35.12	34.07
99232	40.84	46.55	47.33	48.32
99233	15.23	17.37	17.55	17.61
Same date observation/hospital				
99234	28.22	37.22	23.39	41.29
99235	39.46	29.62	24.70	24.22
99236	32.32	33.16	51.90	34.49
Hospital discharge day				
99238	76.93	70.72	69.76	68.49
99239	23.07	29.28	30.24	31.51
Office consultation				
99241	6.23	5.69	10.46	10.69
99242	9.27	8.16	7.16	6.68
99243	11.52	19.93	21.38	17.98
99244	38.09	35.98	33.35	36.22
99245	34.89	30.24	27.66	28.43
Inpatient consultation				
99251	5.57	5.16	4.93	5.08
99252	13.14	12.66	12.36	12.08
99253	28.13	28.86	29.31	30.40
99254	35.70	37.23	37.49	36.61
99255	17.47	16.09	15.90	15.84

NATIONAL DISTRIBUTION OF EVALUATION AND MANAGEMENT CODE SELECTION BY PSYCHIATRISTS (*CONTINUED*)

CODE	NATIONAL DISTRIBUTION 2001, %	NATIONAL DISTRIBUTION 2006, %	NATIONAL DISTRIBUTION 2007, %	NATIONAL DISTRIBUTION 2008, %
Emergency department visit				
99281	11.02	6.40	5.14	4.43
99282	15.27	11.38	12.21	11.62
99283	28.09	28.71	29.66	31.14
99284	19.91	30.89	28.88	32.38
99285	25.71	22.62	24.11	20.43
Initial nursing facility care				
99304		14.55	10.81	11.92
99305		36.56	37.23	34.37
99306		48.89	51.96	53.71
Subsequent nursing facility care				
99307		24.27	21.57	19.32
99308		37.30	38.34	38.65
99309		26.49	27.17	27.58
99310		11.94	12.91	14.45
Nursing facility discharge day				
99315		34.47	23.06	21.71
99316		65.53	76.94	78.29
Domicile/R-home visit, new patient				
99324		7.76	5.45	5.21
99325		17.70	11.91	9.77
99326		26.70	24.54	19.03
99327		17.90	24.38	26.61
99328		29.94	33.73	39.38

NATIONAL DISTRIBUTION OF EVALUATION AND MANAGEMENT CODE SELECTION BY PSYCHIATRISTS (*CONTINUED*)

CODE	NATIONAL DISTRIBUTION 2001, %	NATIONAL DISTRIBUTION 2006, %	NATIONAL DISTRIBUTION 2007, %	NATIONAL DISTRIBUTION 2008, %
Domicile/R-home visit, established patient				
99334		29.02	27.33	22.01
99335		37.85	38.30	35.55
99336		24.72	25.78	34.10
99337		8.41	8.58	8.34
Home visits, new patient				
99341		1.04	0.87	1.48
99342		8.23	3.81	7.97
99343		18.50	16.48	16.55
99344		37.17	31.20	22.80
99345		35.06	47.64	51.20
Home visits, established patient				
99347		10.72	6.02	5.01
99348		34.83	33.95	30.95
99349		39.23	43.68	40.38
99350		15.21	16.34	23.66

Appendix L

American Psychiatric Association CPT Coding Service and Additional Resources

The American Psychiatric Association (APA) maintains a Current Procedural Terminology (CPT) coding service to answer its members' specific coding questions, and the association is actively involved in making sure that members are correctly reimbursed for the services they provide. Working closely with the Committee on RBRVS, Codes, and Reimbursements, the APA's Office of Healthcare Systems and Financing (OHSF) has established a CPT coding service. Because CPT questions are very specific and often very complex, a protocol has been established for queries to ensure that there will be no misunderstanding.

APA members with CPT coding questions should:

1. create an e-mail or memo with their name, APA member number, city, state, phone number, fax number, and e-mail address;
2. state the question or describe the problem thoroughly but succinctly—a short paragraph is usually all that is necessary;
3. include any relevant correspondence from Medicare carriers, insurance companies, or third-party payers;
4. cite any actions that have been taken relating to the problem, for example, calls made or letters written; and
5. send the question to the attention of Rebecca Yowell by e-mail (hsf@psych.org), fax (703-907-1089), or regular mail (Office of Healthcare Systems and Financing, APA, 1000 Wilson Boulevard, Suite 1825, Arlington, VA 22209).

All questions will be answered as quickly as possible.

COURSES/WORKSHOPS

A CPT coding continuing medical education course and a CPT workshop are generally held each year at the APA's annual meeting. Check the APA annual meeting program for more information.

OTHER MEMBERSHIP ORGANIZATIONS

Mental health clinicians who are not members of the APA should contact their own member specialty societies. These organizations may have in place CPT resources similar to those available through the APA. Organizations that may be of interest include the following:

- American Nurses Association: www.nursingworld.org; 800-274-4262
- American Psychiatric Nurses Association: www.apna.org; 866-243-2443
- American Psychological Association: www.apa.org; 800-374-2721 or 202-336-5500
- National Association of Social Workers: www.naswdc.org; 202-336-8200

Appendix M

Medicare Carriers and Administrative Contractors

The Medicare program is in the process of making a transition from Medicare Carriers to Medicare Administrative Contractors. Medicare Carriers oversee Part B for specific states. The contractors will eventually oversee both Parts A and B for all of the 15 jurisdictions that the Centers for Medicare and Medicaid Services (CMS) has designated. The transition was to be complete in 2010, but a number of the contracts have been protested, so the process has been delayed indefinitely. Unfortunately, it has been very difficult to get contact information on the Administrative Contractors. Hopefully by the time you read this, the information will be available on the CMS Web site.

As we go to press, Medicare Administrative Contractors are in place in 9 of the 15 jurisdictions. The CMS Web site should have the most current listings for Medicare carriers and contractors, which can be accessed at

https://www. cms.gov/MedicareContractingReform/Downloads/Primary/ABMACJurisdictionFactSheets.pdf

J1—California, Hawaii, and Nevada
Palmetto GBA
Columbia, SC
http://palmettogba.com/palmetto/palmetto.nsf/DocsCat/Home

J3—Arizona, Montana, North Dakota, South Dakota, Utah, and Wyoming
Noridian Administrative Services
Fargo, ND
https://www.noridianmedicare.com/

J4—Colorado, New Mexico, Oklahoma, and Texas
Trailblazer Health Enterprises
Dallas, TX
http://www.trailblazerhealth.com/

J5—Iowa, Kansas, Missouri, and Nebraska
Wisconsin Physician Services
Madison, WI
http://www.wpsmedicare.com/

J9—Florida, Puerto Rico, and the U.S. Virgin Islands
First Coast Service Options
Jacksonville, FL
http://medicare.fcso.com

J10—Alabama, Georgia, and Tennessee
Cahaba GBA (Government Benefit Administrators)
Birmingham, AL
http://cahabagba.com

J12—Delaware, District of Columbia, Maryland, New Jersey, Northern Virginia, and Pennsylvania
Highmark Medicare Services
Camp Hill, PA
http://www.highmarkmedicareservices.com/

J13—Connecticut and New York
National Government Services
Syracuse, NY
http://www.ngsmedicare.com/ngsmedicare/HomePage.aspx

J14—Maine, Massachusetts, New Hampshire, Rhode Island, and Vermont
National Heritage Insurance Corporation
Hingham, MA
http://www.medicarenhic.com/

Appendix N

Centers for Medicare and Medicaid Services Regional Offices

The Centers for Medicare and Medicaid Services (CMS), which is located in Baltimore, Maryland, has 10 regional offices that oversee the new Medicare Administrative Contractors and the remaining Medicare Part B carriers and Part A fiscal intermediaries in the states included in their regions. These regional offices also oversee the federal component of the Medicaid programs and children's health insurance plans in these states. The latest information on the regional offices, staff responsibilities, and e-mail addresses and phone numbers for staff can be found at http://www.cms.hhs.gov/regionaloffices/. Information about each office can be accessed under "Downloads" at the bottom of the page.

REGION I: BOSTON

States covered: Connecticut, Maine, Massachusetts, New Hampshire, Rhode Island, and Vermont
Address: Office of the Regional Administrator, JFK Federal Building, Suite 2325, Boston, MA 02203-0003
Phone: 617-565-1188

REGION II: NEW YORK

States covered: New York and New Jersey, as well as the U.S. Virgin Islands and Puerto Rico
Address: Office of the Regional Administrator, Jacob K. Javits Federal Building, 26 Federal Plaza, Room 3811, New York, NY 10278-0063
Phone: 212-616-2205

REGION III: PHILADELPHIA

States covered: Delaware, Maryland, Pennsylvania, Virginia, West Virginia, and the District of Columbia
Address: Office of the Regional Administrator, Public Ledger Building, Suite 216, 150 South Independence Mall West, Philadelphia, PA 19106
Phone: 215-861-4140

REGION IV: ATLANTA

States covered: Alabama, Florida, Georgia, Kentucky, Mississippi, North Carolina, South Carolina, and Tennessee
Address: Office of the Regional Administrator, Atlanta Federal Center, 61 Forsyth Street, SW, Suite 4T20, Atlanta, GA 30303-8909
Phone: 404-562-7150

REGION V: CHICAGO

States covered: Illinois, Indiana, Michigan, Minnesota, Ohio, and Wisconsin
Address: Office of the Regional Administrator, 233 North Michigan Avenue, Suite 600, Chicago, IL 60601
Phone: 312-886-6432

REGION VI: DALLAS

States covered: Arkansas, Louisiana, New Mexico, Oklahoma, and Texas
Address: Office of the Regional Administrator, 1301 Young Street, Suite 714, Dallas, TX 75202
Phone: 214-767-6427

REGION VII: KANSAS CITY

States covered: Iowa, Kansas, Missouri, and Nebraska
Address: Office of the Regional Administrator, 601 East 12th Street, Suite 235, Kansas City, MO 64106
Phone: 816-426-5233

REGION VIII: DENVER

States covered: Colorado, Montana, North Dakota, South Dakota, Utah, and Wyoming
Address: Office of the Regional Administrator, 1600 Broadway, Suite 700, Denver, CO 80202
Phone: 303-844-2111

REGION IX: SAN FRANCISCO

States covered: Arizona, California, Hawaii, and Nevada, as well as the territories of American Samoa, Guam, and the Commonwealth of the Northern Mariana Islands
Address: Office of the Regional Administrator, 90 7th Street, Suite 5-300, San Francisco, CA 94103-6706
Phone: 415-744-3501

REGION X: SEATTLE

States covered: Alaska, Idaho, Oregon, and Washington
Address: Office of the Regional Administrator, 2201 Sixth Avenue, Suite 801, Seattle, WA 98121
Phone: 206-615-2306

Index

Page numbers printed in **boldface** type refer to page numbers in the appendixes. Page numbers printed in *italic* type refer to text page numbers in tabular material.

Albaum-Feinstein, Dr. Andrea L., 93
Alzheimer's disease, Medicare and, 19
AMA. *See* American Medical Association
American Academy of Child and Adolescent
　　Psychiatry, **101**
American Hospital Association, **101**
American Medical Association (AMA)
　　CPT coding system and, 1
　　CPT Editorial Panel and, **101**
　　Healthcare Professionals Advisory Committee
　　　　(HCPAC), 1, **101**
　　House of Delegates, 1
American Nurses Association, **101, 178**
American Psychiatric Association (APA), 4, **101**
　　CPT coding service, **177–178**
　　Office of Healthcare Systems and Financing,
　　　　5, **177–178**
American Psychiatric Nurses Association, 4, **178**
American Psychological Association, **101, 178**
APA. *See* American Psychiatric Association
Aphasia, 25
Appendixes, structure of CPT manual and, 3–4
Appointments, Medicare policy of, 80
Assisted living facility, 97

Balanced Budget Act of 1997, 76
Balanced Budget Refinement Act of 1999, 75
Behavior change interventions, codes for, *32*

Blue Cross/Blue Shield Association, 1, 74, **101**
Boston Diagnostic Aphasia Examination, 25
Braun, Dr. Peter, 74
Bundling, of services, 94

California Blue Shield, 74
California Medical Association, 74
Case management services, codes for, 58
CC. *See* Chief complaint
CCI. *See* Correct Coding Initiative
Centers for Medicare and Medicaid Services
　　(CMS), 1, 71, 91, **101, 103, 179**
　　guidelines for evaluation and management
　　　　services, **115–128**
Central nervous system assessments/tests, codes
　　for, 24–26
Chief complaint (CC), 34
　　documentation, **118**
　　elements required for, *35*
　　patient history taking and, *38*
Claims management and review, 85–86
　　submission of claims, 93–94
Clinical nurse specialists (CNSs), Medicare
　　payment policies and, 76
Clinical psychologists, Medicare payment
　　policies and, 76
Clinical social workers (CSWs), Medicare
　　payment policies and, 76

CMS. *See* Centers for Medicare and Medicaid Services

CNSs. *See* Clinical nurse specialists

Codes

accuracy of, 91–96

Categories II and III, 3

changing requirements and, 95

place of service (POS) codes for Medicare, **113–114**

selection of, 92–93

Codes, reference to specific

90801, 12–13, 27, 28, *64, 65, 67, 75*, 98, 99, **164**

90802, 13–14, 27, *64, 67*, **164**

90804, 15, *64, 65*, **164**

90805, 15, *64*, **164**

90806, 15, *64, 65*, **164**

90807, 15, *64*, **112, 164**

90808, 15, *64, 65* **164**

90809, 15, *64*, **164**

90810, 15, **164**

90811, 15, **164**

90812, 15, **164**

90813, 15, **164**

90814, 15, **164**

90815, 15, **164**

90816, 16, **164**

90817, 16, *67*, **164**

90818, 16, **164**

90819, 16, *67*, **164**

90821, 16, **164**

90822, 16, **164**

90823, 16, **164**

90824, 16, **164**

90826, 16, **164**

90827, 16, **164**

90828, 16, **165**

90829, 16, **165**

90845, 16–17, *65*, **165**

90846, 17, *65*, **165**

90847, 17–18, *65*, **165**

90849, 18, **165**

90853, 18, **165**

90857, 18–19, **165**

90862, 19, *19*, 27, 60, *64, 65, 67*, 97–98, **155, 165**

90865, 20, **165**

90870, 20, **165**

90875, 20, **165**

90876, 20, **165**

90880, 20–21, **165**

90882, 21, **165**

90885, 21, **165**

90887, 21–22, **165**

90889, 22, **165**

90899, 22, 28, **165**

90901, **165**

90911, **165**

90935, **165**

90937, **165**

95805, 23

95806, 23

95807, 23

95808, 24

95810, 24

95811, 24

96101, 24, **166**

96102, 24, **166**

96103, 25, **166**

96105, 25, **166**

96110, 25, **166**

96111, 25, **166**

96116, 25, **166**

96118, 25

96119, 26, **166**

96120, 26, **166**

96125, 26, **166**

96150, 27, **166**

96151, 27, **166**

96152, 27, **166**

96153, 27, **166**

96154, 27, **166**

96155, 27, **166**

96201, **166**

96202, **166**

96203, **166**

96204, **166**

99201, *32*, 47, *64, 65*, **172**

99202, *32*, 47, *64, 65*, **172**

99203, *32*, 47, *64*, **129, 172**

99204, *32, 47, 64*, **172**

99205, *32*, 47, *64*, **129–130, 172**

99211, 48, *65, 66*, 98, **167, 172**

99212, *19*, 48, *64, 65, 66*, 98, **167, 172**

99213, 48, *64, 65, 66*, 98, **130, 167, 172**

99214, 48, *66*, **167, 172**

99215, 48, **167, 172**

99217, *32*, 48, **167**

99218, *32*, 48, **167, 172**

99219, *32*, 49, **167, 172**

99220, *32*, 49, **167, 172**

99221, *32,,* 33, 45–46, 49, 60, *67*, 98, 99, **130, 167, 172**

99222, *32*, 33, 49, *67*, 98, 99, **131, 167, 172**

99223, 12, *32*, 33, 34, 44–45, 49, *67*, 98, 99, **167, 172**

99231, *32*, 50, **133, 167, 173**

99232, *32*, 50, *67*, **167, 173**

99233, *32*, 50, *67*, **167, 173**

99234, **173**

99235, **167, 173**

99236, **167, 173**

99238, *32*, 50, *67*, **167, 173**

99239, *32*, 50, *67*, **167, 173**

99241, *32*, 51, **167, 173**

99242, *32*, 51, **167, 173**

99243, *32*, 51, **167, 173**

99244, *32*, 51, **134, 167, 173**

99245, *32*, 51, **134–135, 173**

99251, *32*, 51, **168, 173**

99252, *32*, 52, **168, 173**

99253, *32*, 52, **168, 173**

99254, *32*, 52, **135, 168, 173**

99255, *32*, 52, **136, 168, 173**

99281, *32*, 52, **168, 174**

99282, *32*, 52, **168, 174**

99283, *32*, 52, **168, 174**

99284, *32*, 52, **168, 174**

99285, *32*, 52, **168, 174**

99286, *32*

99287, *32*

99288, *32*, **168**

99291, **168**

99292, **168**

99304, *32*, 53, *68*, **168, 174**

99305, *32*, 53, *68*, **168, 174**

99306, *32*, 53, **168, 174**

99307, *32*, 54, *69*, **168, 174,**

99308, *32*, 54, *69*, **168, 174**

99309, *32*, 54, *69*, **168, 174**

99310, *32*, 54, *69*, **168, 174**

99315, *32*, 54, **168, 174**

99316, *32*, 54, **168, 174**

99318, *32*, 54, **168**

99324, *32*, 55, **169, 174**

99325, *32*, 55, **169, 174**

99326, *32*, 55, **169, 174**

99327, *32*, 55, **169, 174**

99328, *32*, 55, **169, 174**

99334, *32*, 56, **169, 175**

99335, *32*, 56, **169, 175**

99336, *32*, 56, **169, 175**

99337, *32*, 56, **169, 175**

99339, **169**

99340, **169**

99341, *32*, 56, **169, 175**

99342, *32*, 57, **169, 175**

99343, *32*, 57, **169, 175**

99344, *32*, 57, **169, 175**

99345, *32*, 57, **169, 175**

99347, *32*, 57, **169, 175**

99348, *32*, 57, **169, 175**

99349, *32*, 58, **169, 175**

99350, *32*, 58, **169, 175**

99355, **169**

99356, **169**

99357, **169**

99358, **169**

99366, *32*, 58

99367, *32*, 58

99406, *32*, 58

99407, *32*, 58

99408, *32*, 58

99409, *32*, 58

99441, 28, *32*, 58

99442, 28, *32*, 58

99443, 28, *32*, 58

99444, 28, *32*, 58

99450, *32*, 59

99455, *32*, 59

99456, *32*, 59

M0064, *19*, 23, *64, 65*

Cognitive performance testing, code for, 26

Commercial insurance. *See* Health insurance

Complications, as risks, 41, *42*

Conjoint psychotherapy, 17–18

Consultations, 60, **139**

   codes for, *32*, 50–52

   codes for inpatient, 51–52

   codes for office or other outpatient consultations, 51, **134–135**

   follow-up care after, 68, *68*

   initial inpatient, **135–136**

   inpatient, codes for, **173**

   for inpatient services, 68

   templates

      for attending consultant physician psychiatry evaluation, **151–154**

      for psychiatric consultation, **150**

Coordination of care, documentation of, **127–128**

Correct Coding Initiative (CCI), 77

Counseling

   documentation of an encounter dominated by coordination of care of, **127–128**

   E/M codes and, 31

CPT. *See* Current procedural terminology

CSWs. *See* Clinical social workers

Current procedural terminology (CPT), 1–5

    access to current edition, 5

    accurate coding and, 91–96

    Advisory Committee, 1, **101–102**

    AMA Editorial Panel, **101**

    Categories II and III, codes for, 3

    coding service, 5, **177–178**

    courses/workshops, **178**

    Editorial Panel, 1, **103**

    evaluation and management codes.
        See Evaluation and management (E/M)
        codes

    instructions for primary classes of, 4

    insurance companies and, 5

    major clinical sections, 2–3

    process for requesting updates of, **102–103**

    structure of, 2–5

    verification of, 94

Custodial care services, codes for, *32*, 55–56

Date of service, **139**

Decision making, 39, **139**

    amount and/or complexity of data to be
        reviewed, *41*

    determination of level, 43

    documentation of medical, **124–127**

    elements and type of, 43, *43*

    types of, *43*

Developmental testing, codes for, 25

Diagnoses and management options, 41, *41*

    documentation, **125–127**

Diagnosis-related groups (DRGs), 73–74

Diagnostic tests

    amount and/or complexity of data to be
        reviewed, *41*

    risks, 41, *42*

Discharge services

    codes for hospital discharge services, 50, *67*,
        173

    codes for nursing facility services, 54, **174**

Disclosure, **108**

Documentation, **138, 139**

    accuracy of, 7–8

    of an encounter dominated by counseling or
        coordination of care, **127–128**

    audit liability and, 7

    changing requirements and, 95

    importance of, **115**

    of medical decision making, **124–127**

    of medical records, 9

    of number of diagnoses or management
        options, **125–127**

    principles of, 9–10

    of psychiatric service codes, 10

    selection of codes and, 7

    of services, 93

    templates for, **141–155**

Domiciliary care services

    codes for, *32*, 55–56

    codes for established patient, 56

    codes for new patient, 55

DRGs. *See* Diagnosis-related groups

ECT. *See* Electroconvulsive therapy

Electroconvulsive therapy (ECT)

    codes for, 20

    consent form template, **160**

    memory problems with, **159**

    number of treatments, **158**

    patient information, **157**

    procedure, **157–158**

    record template, **161**

    recovery, **158**

    risks of, **158–159**

Electronic medical records (EMRs), 91

E/M. *See* Evaluation and management codes;
    Evaluation and management services

E-mail, code for, 28

Emergency department services, 98–99

    codes for, *32*, 52–53, **174**

EMRs. *See* Electronic medical records

Environmental intervention, for medical
    management purposes, 21

Established patient

    codes for, 47–48

    codes for home visits, **174**

    office visit, **130, 172**

Evaluation and management (E/M) codes

    for case management services, 58

    codes most likely to be used by psychiatrists, *32*

    coding and documentation for specific clinical
        settings, 63–69

    for consultations, 50–52

    descriptor review and instructions, 33

    determination of complexity of medical
        decision making, 39–43

    determination of extent of work required,
        34–39

    determination of performing the
        examination, 39

for domiciliary, rest home, or custodial care
services, 55–56
for emergency department services, 52–53
history of, 29–31
for home services, 56–58
for hospital inpatient services, 49–50
for hospital observational services, 48–49
level of service selection, 31–43
national distribution of code selection by
psychiatrists, **171–175**
for nursing facility services, 53–54, 68–69, *68,
69*
for office or other outpatient services, 47–48
overview, 3
for preventive medicine services, 58–59
requirements for key components of service, 34
selection of appropriate level of service, 44–46,
92–93
for special evaluation and management
services, 59
terminology explained, 30–31
vignettes for, **129–136**
who may use, 59
for work-related or medical disability
evaluation services, 59
Evaluation and management (E/M) services
CMS guidelines for, **115–128**
documentation of, **116–128**
examination, **121–127**
history, **117–121**
Examinations
documentation of, **21–124**
multi-system documentation, **123–124**
single-organ documentation, **122–123**
single-system other than psychiatry, **123–124**

Family psychotherapy
multiple-family group psychotherapy, 18
with the patient present (conjoint
psychotherapy), 17–18
without the patient present, 17
Fees
computing fees for Medicare, *64, 67, 68, 69, 75,
75,* 81, **163–169**
physician fee schedule, **163–169**

Gordy, Dr. Tracy, 1, **101**
Group psychotherapy
interactive, 18–19
multiple-family, 18
other than of a multiple-family group, 18

Harvard School of Public Health, 74
HCFA. *See* Health Care Financing
Administration
HCPAC. *See* Healthcare Professionals Advisory
Committee
Health and behavior assessment/intervention,
codes for, 26–27
Healthcare Common Procedure Coding System, 2
Health Care Financing Administration (HCFA),
29. *See also* Centers for Medicare and
Medicaid Services
Medicare and, 74
Medicare teaching-physician rules, 77
Healthcare Professionals Advisory Committee
(HCPAC), **101**
Health insurance. *See also* Medicare
changes in the healthcare system, 83–84
claims management and review, 85–86, 89
commercial insurance issues, 83–89
health maintenance organizations (HMOs)
and, 89
managed care companies and, 89
negative impact and, 84
oversight, 86
problems with, 89
reimbursement of, 95
role of private in the medical system, 83
strategies for dealing with insurance
companies, 86–88
developing and maintaining relationships
with insurance companies, 86–87
when things go wrong, 87–88
Health Insurance Association of America, 1, **101**
Health Insurance Portability and Accountability
Act of 1966 (HIPAA), 2, 91, 93, **105–109**
minimum disclosure and, **108**
overview, **105–106**
patients' rights and, **107–108**
physician compliance and, **108–109**
Privacy Rule, **107–109**
psychotherapy notes and, **108**
requirements, 10
Security Rule, **109**
Transactions Rule, **106–107**
Health maintenance organizations (HMOs), 89
HIPAA. *See* Health Insurance Portability and
Accountability Act
History of present illness (HPI), 34, **138**
documentation, **119**
elements required for, *35*
patient history taking and, *38*

HMO Act of 1973, 83
HMOs. *See* Health maintenance organizations
Home services
    codes for, *32,* 56–58
    codes for established patient, 57–58, **174**
    codes for new patient, 56–57, **174**
Hospital records
    interpretation or explanation of results of
        medical examinations and procedures,
        21–22
    psychiatric evaluation of, 21
Hospital visits, 60
    acute hospital and partial hospital services
        using E/M codes, 66–67
    alternative coding possibilities for adult hospi-
        tal and partial hospital services, 68, *67*
    codes for emergency department services, *32,*
        52–53, **174**
    codes for hospital discharge services, 50
    codes for inpatient services, 49–50
    codes for observational services, *32,* 48–49
    codes for subsequent hospital care, 50
    discharge codes, *67*
    initial hospital care, codes for, 66, *67,* **172,**
    inpatient services, **130–133**
        codes for, *32*
    same day observation, codes for, **173**
    subsequent or partial care, *67, 67,* **133–134,**
        173
HPI. *See* History of present illness
Hsaio, Dr. William, 74
Hypnotherapy, code for, 20

ICD codes, verification of, 94
Information technology, 91
Injections, Medicare payment policies and, 75–76
Inpatient services
    codes for, *32*
    consultations, 68
Insurance companies. *See also* Health insurance
    developing and maintaining relationships
        with, 86–87
    problems with, 89
    procedures listed in CPT and, 5

Kaiser Family Foundation, 83

LCD. *See* Local coverage determination
Legislation
    Balanced Budget Act of 1997, 76
    Balanced Budget Refinement Act of 1999, 75

Health Insurance Portability and
    Accountability Act of 1966 (HIPAA), 2,
    91, 93, **105–109**
    HMO Act of 1973, 83
Local coverage determination (LCD), Medicare
    and, 78–79

Managed care organization (MCO), 84, 89
Management options, risks and, 41, *42*
MCO. *See* Managed care companies
Medicaid, 2, 83
    centers by region, **181–183**
Medical decision making. *See* Decision making
Medical disability evaluation services, codes for,
    59
Medically Unlikely Edits (MUEs), 77
Medical records, documentation principles of, 9,
    116
Medical team conferences, codes for, 58
Medicare, 2, 71–81. *See also* Health insurance
    advance beneficiary notice and, 79
    Advantage Plans, 71–72
    advantages, 80
    Alzheimer's disease and, 19
    carriers, 71
    carriers and administrative contractors by
        state, **179–180**
    centers by region, **181–183**
    computing fees and, 75, *75*
    consultation codes and, 61
    Correct Coding Initiative (CCI) and, 77
    deductible/copayment and, 81
    E/M codes and, 29
    fees, *64, 67,* 68, 69, 81, **163–169**
    fiscal intermediaries and, 71
    history of, 71–72
    limiting charges for services not covered by, 81
    local coverage determination (LCD) and,
        78–79
    Medically Unlikely Edits (MUEs), 77
    nonparticipating providers and, 80
    nonreimbursement issues, 21–22
    opting out of and private contracting, 79–80
    outpatient mental health treatment limitation
        and, 72
    participation/nonparticipation in, 73
    payment policies, 75–78
    physician payment reform of, 73–74
    physician reimbursement system, **103**
    place of services (POS) codes for, **113–114**
    policy for missed appointments, 80

reimbursement and, 95–96
relative value units, **163–169**
residents and, 99
as secondary payer, 78
teaching-physician rules, 77, 98
in transition, 71
Medicare Administrative Contractors, **179**
Medicare Advantage plan, 80
Medicare RBRVS: The Physicians' Guide, 74
Mental status examination, 39, *40*
checklist, 61
Modifiers, **111–112**
documentation requirements of, **112**
mandated services, **112**
reduced services, **112**
Morbidity, risks and, 41, *42, 43*
Mortality, risks and, 41, *42, 43*
Musculoskeletal system, content and
documentation requirements for, *40*

Narcosynthesis, code for, 20
National Association of Social Workers, 4–5, **101, 178**
Neurobehavioral status examination, 25
Neuropsychological testing, codes for, 26
New patient, **172**
codes for, 47
codes for home visits, **174**
defined, 30
initial hospital care, codes for, 66, *67*
office visit, **129–130**
selection of appropriate level of service, 44
Nixon, President Richard, 83
Nonphysicians, Medicare payment policies and, 76
Nonpsychiatric mental health services, 23–27
NPs. *See* Nurse-practitioners
Nurse-practitioners (NPs), Medicare payment policies and, 76
Nursing facility services
codes for, *32,* 53–54, **174**
codes for discharge services, 54, **174**
codes for initial care, 53
codes for new or established patient, 68, *68*
codes for subsequent care, 54, 68, *69, 69*

Observation care, **172**
Office of Healthcare Systems and Financing (OHSF) (American Psychiatric Association), 5, **177–178**

Office visit
brief, 23
codes for, *32,* 47–48
for established patient—return visits, 66, **130**
initial visit—diagnostic interview, codes for, 63, *64*
for monitoring or change drug prescriptions, 23
for new patient, **129–130, 172**
office or other outpatient evaluation and management services, codes for, 66, *66*
OHSF. *See* Office of Healthcare Systems and Financing
Outpatient mental health treatment limitation, 72
Outpatient services
codes for, *32,* 47–48
split management between physician and nonphysician providers, codes for, 65, *65*
Oversight, 86

PAs. *See* Physician assistants
Past, family, and/or social history (PFSH), 36–37, 39
documentation, **120–121**
elements required for, 34, *35*
patient history taking and, *38*
Patient history
documentation of, 37, 39
names, **139**
taking, *38*
Patient physical exam, **138**
Patient services, 92
Patients' rights, **107**
Payers, **116**
PFSH. *See* Past, family, and/or social history
Pharmacological management, 97
brief office visit for monitoring or changing drug prescriptions, 23
codes for, 19–20, 60, 64, *64*
template for, **155**
Physician assistants (PAs), Medicare payment policies and, 76
Physician Payment Review Commission, 74
Physicians
compliance with HIPAA, **108–109**
signature, **139**
templates
for attending physician admission note, **142–146**
for attending physician subsequent care, **147–149**

Physician services
  codes for non-face-to-face services, *32*
  face-to-face services, 44
Physicians' Current Procedural Terminology
    (AMA, 1966). *See* Current procedural
    terminology
Place of service (POS) codes, for Medicare, **113–114**
Polysomnography, 24
Preventive medicine services
  codes for, 58–59
  codes for counseling risk factor reduction and
      behavior change intervention, 58
  codes for non-face-to-face services, 58
  codes for on-line medical evaluation, 59
Privacy rule, of the Health Insurance Portability
    and Accountability Act (HIPAA), **106–107**
Professional societies, health insurance and, 89
Psychiatric diagnostic or evaluative interview
    procedures, 12–14
  presenting problems, 41, *42*
Psychiatric evaluation, *40*
  content and documentation requirements for,
      40
  documentation, 9
  template for attending consultant physician
      psychiatry evaluation, **151–154**
  template for psychiatric consultation, **150**
Psychiatric service codes, 60
  documentation, 10
  unlisted code, 22
Psychiatric status, preparation of report of, 22
Psychiatric therapeutic procedures, 14–19
Psychiatrists, national distribution of evaluation
    and management code selection by, **171–175**
Psychoanalysis, codes for, 16–17
Psychophysiological therapy, codes for, 20
Psychotherapy, notes and, **108**
Psychotherapy codes, 14–19, 97
  in an inpatient hospital, partial hospital, or
      residential care facility, 16
  in an office or other outpatient facility, 15–16
  individual codes for, 64, *64*
  interactive, 16

RBBRVS. *See* Resource-Based Relative Value Scale
Reimbursement, 95
Relative value units (RVUs), **163–169**
Residents, Medicare and, 99
Resource-Based Relative Value Scale (RBBRVS),
    72, **103**
  Medicare payment system and, 81

Rest home services, codes for, *32,* 55–56
Review of symptoms (ROS), 34, 35–36
  checklist, 60
  documentation, **119–120**
  elements required for, *35*
  patient history taking and, *38*
Risk, **128**
ROS. *See* Review of symptoms
Ross Information Processing Assessment, 26
RUC. *See* RVS Update Committee
RVS Update Committee (RUC), **103**
RVUs. *See* Relative value units

Security Rule, of the Health Insurance Portability
    and Accountability Act (HIPAA), **109**
Single system psychiatric examination, content
    and documentation requirements, *40*
Sleep testing, codes for, 23–24
Special evaluation and management services,
    codes for, 59

Teaching-physician, Medicare rules and,
    77, 98
Team conference services, codes for, *32,* 60
Telephone
  codes for, 28
  Medicare payment policies and, 75
  psychotherapy provided by, 28
Templates
  for documentation, **141–155**
  ECT consent form, **160**
  ECT record, **161**
Therapeutic procedures, 9
Time, selection of level of service and, 45, *46*
Time-based codes, **139**
Transactions Rule, of the Health Insurance
    Portability and Accountability Act (HIPAA),
    1–2, **106–107**
Treatment plan, 9

Unbundling, of services, 94
U.S. Congress, 74
U.S. Department of Health and Human Services
    (DHHS), **101, 105**

Verification, of codes, 94
Vital signs, measurement of, *40*

Work-related disability evaluation services, codes
    for, 59
Workshops, on CPT coding, **178**